Currents in American Medicine

A Developmental View of Medical Care and Education

Currents in

A Developmental View of

A Commonwealth Fund Book

American Medicine

Medical Care and Education

Julius B. Richmond, M.D.

Foreword by Ward Darley, M.D.

Harvard University Press Cambridge, Massachusetts

To Rhee

Foreword
Ward Darley, M.D.

The tempo and the thrust of events that have shaped the American medical establishment since 1900 give a particular timeliness to *Currents in American Medicine*. The author focuses on the most important of the positive and negative factors that have resulted in the present educational, research, and service aspects of today's system, or, as Anne Somers has recently suggested, "non-system," of medicine.

The book has been written so that those concerned with service or with research or with education may perceive the stream of events pursuing different courses, accelerating in pace or seeming to stand still as it is acted upon by various internal and external factors. The realization for all readers should be that we have a medical establishment which has had a Topsy-like growth to tremendous size and complexity, which is characterized by ideas and plans that were born before their time, by clashes between vested and perceived interests resulting in expediencies and compromises that have constituted obstacles to progress lasting years on end, and by failure to recognize that what may be considered progress in one area can cause almost insoluble problems in another.

For example, a thoughtful reader will find that in the decade 1910–1920, the curricular standardization that resulted from the recommendations of Abraham Flexner was the only way to improve the then chaotic state of physician education. Yet it will also be clear that after this standardization had served its purpose, with very few exceptions its resulting rigidities, aided and abetted by the interests of specialism, stifled badly needed curricular innovation. Now, fifty years later, curricular innovation is finally beginning to appear.

But to decry specialism as something evil would be unfair, because specialism is the only way that the human mind and the human world can make use of the tremendous increases in knowledge that have resulted from the growth in supported research during the past twenty-five years. No one human being can be expected to encompass more than a limited portion of this knowledge; particularly in medicine, new knowledge has had to be broken down into learnable parts.

It seems inevitable that both knowledge and specialism will continue to increase. But in medicine, specialism has been the result of the fragmentation of knowledge, and the result of specialism has been the fragmentation of medical care. In the process there has been an increasing emphasis upon the episodic care of the manifestations of disease and a decreasing concern for the person in whom the disease is present. (This fragmentation of care is emphasized by the entrenched practice of paying for service piece by piece.) Lack of concern for the entire person is influenced by socio-economic factors such as urbanization and crowding and by the twin factors of homogenization and anonymity that can so easily result.

It may be that this pendulum has reached the end of its swing. For recently, in response to the interest of private citizens in improving medical care and in response to various pieces of federal legislation (the most important listed in Dr. Richmond's book), we have begun to see islands of innovation. Gradually our health resources are being employed in new ways to develop person-centered, continuing, comprehensive care. As Dr. Richmond reviews the history behind these innovations, the tragedy of the lags between ideas and action and the reasons for these lags at once become apparent. To appreciate this point, all the reader has to do is review the recommendations of the 1932 report of the Committee on the Costs of Medical Care and the reasons for the submergence of this report; then note the old recommendations that are emerging today under the name of innovation. Or the reader can review the immediate post-World War II developments, the Hill-Burton Hospital Construc-

tion Act and the federal support of medical research, which
would of necessity call for rapidly increasing numbers and kinds
of health and medical personnel. Yet it was another fifteen to
twenty years before anything was done to enable the educational
establishment to take positive action on this problem.

Dr. Richmond's book underscores the urgent need for lay-
man and professional alike to understand the ins and outs
of the nation's growing and changing medical world. Dr.
Richmond calls attention to the possible role of the Regional
Medical Programs and Comprehensive Health Planning legislation in providing coordination and facilitating communication. He particularly hopes that the new Board of Medicine of
the National Academy of Sciences will develop into an acceptable and durable agency for over-all national health planning.

In his final chapter Dr. Richmond clearly points out the priorities that must obtain if the future effectiveness of American
medicine is to reach anything like its full potential. He notes
that years ago Dr. Alan Gregg began calling attention to the
consequences of ignoring the importance of multiple causation.
Today, with little control over the pollution of air, water,
and soil; with advertising cleverly plugging for the pleasures of
tobacco and alcohol; and with tensions mounting in response to
the complexities of life in home, school, church, and job, it is
time to heed Dr. Gregg's warning and give due consideration to
the long-range consequences of our actions. If thought is given
to the future directions of medicine as well as to the present care
of manifest disease, the result will be a dedication to the discov-
ery and management of asymptomatic disease and to the pro-
motion of comprehensive health services.

The achievement of these goals will require something like
the community organization set forth by Dr. Richmond. We can
no longer expect to cope with the increasing complexities of
health and disease and their economic contingencies without
plans and programs that can coordinate education and research
in the interests of developing the broad spectrum of services required for this nation's future strength and effectiveness.

Preface

Few efforts have been made to review historically the rapid changes which have been taking place in the field of health over the past several decades. It is therefore the objective of this presentation to attempt a historical analysis of the evolution of medical services, education, and research in the United States since 1900 and, on the basis of this analysis, to raise questions for the future development of medicine as an institution in our society. Although many of the issues dealt with lend themselves to a more detailed analysis, such an analysis has not been feasible in this volume.

I have made an effort to avoid the jargon of the health professions in order to interest the general reader without detracting from the book's interest for professional persons. In addition, no effort has been made to utilize the language of the social sciences. However, this presentation may be considered as an institutional case history which social scientists may wish to analyze. As is true of any historical presentation, the interpretation of data is personal.

I am indebted to many colleagues who have influenced my development in ways too numerous to mention. A few must be mentioned specifically: Dr. Joseph English, Dr. Sterling D. Garrard, Mrs. Lisbeth Bamberger Schorr, Mr. Jule Sugarman and Dr. Howard Weinberger have been helpful, stimulating, and critical. I am grateful to Mr. R. Sargent Shriver for his leadership and courage in affording me opportunities to translate knowledge into programs. It is also necessary to express appreciation to the writers of the "News and Comment" section of *Science* for their consistently fine reporting; it is difficult to acknowledge all their contributions individually when writing on current scientific issues.

I am deeply grateful to Miss Dorothy Rowden for her editorial suggestions and to Mrs. Sylvia Churgin, who has provided valuable library assistance. To Mrs. Marjorie Huntley, Miss Maxine King, and Mrs. Margaret Menzel it is a pleasure to express again my deep appreciation for their skillful secretarial assistance.

State University of New York   Julius B. Richmond, M.D.
Syracuse, New York   Dean, The College of Medicine
August, 1968

Table of Contents

Illustrations

Currents in American Medicine

A Developmental View of Medical Care and Education

1 The Educational Revolution and the Guild

Establishment (1900–1940)

Trends in Medical Education

At the turn of the century, scientific advances were beginning to have a significant impact on medical education and medical care. Advances in the natural sciences and the increasing availability and applications of the compound microscope fostered the development of pathology, bacteriology, physiology, pharmacology, and biochemistry as sciences basic to the study of medicine. New knowledge in physics and chemistry changed the nature of medical practice through the development of x-ray examinations, electrocardiography, and laboratory examinations of body fluids.

These scientific developments presented medicine and medical education with certain alternatives. First, medical education could go on, as it had in the nineteenth century, training large numbers of physicians through a network of medical schools, many of which were privately owned and managed. This system had produced a favorable physician-population ratio; the relatively large numbers of physicians assured a reasonable distribution to rural as well as urban areas. Medical education was mainly in the hands of practitioners of medicine and reflected the struggles and rivalries of individuals and groups. For example, if a resourceful and able physician was dissatisfied with his fate in one school, he could go off and organize one of his own—and he often did. The history of this period is replete with colorful figures who were itinerants in medical education and who established a string of medical schools in the course of their migrations.

2

It was beyond the resources of most of the proprietary schools to encompass the new scientific developments—for they meant the addition of laboratory instruction, clinical clerkships, and teaching hospitals and the expansion of the trend toward a full-time faculty. The dynamically evolving society in the midst of its industrial revolution seemed ready for the study and reorganization of professional education and services; it did not appear to be willing to wait for the incorporation of scientific advances through the continuance of a large number of medical schools heavily oriented toward a nonscientific training of practitioners with the hope of gradually upgrading the quality of these schools over a period of years. (It may be noted that this was the direction of Soviet medicine following the revolution. Many physicians were trained in medical schools with little research orientation, but the consumer need having been met to a considerable extent, there are now—some fifty years later —many efforts directed at improving the quality of the educational and research programs.)

The second alternative, attempting to improve rapidly all the existing schools, did not seem realistic in terms of available scientific personnel and other resources. The third alternative, the introduction of standards and accrediting processes which would make it impossible for many of these schools to survive, gradually evolved. The catalyst for this development was the Flexner Report of 1910, which presents a detailed account of the state of medical education and practice during the first decade of this century.[1] People have questioned why the study was undertaken at this time. Although the reasons are probably multiple, the most direct explanation is that the Carnegie Foundation for the Advancement of Teaching was then concerned about the state of all professional education. The medical profession seemed to be more ready and willing (particularly through the support of members of the Council on Medical Education of the American Medical Association) than other professional groups; the Foundation therefore elected to proceed with the study of medical education.

The Flexner Report has been widely recognized as one of the most significant developments in American medical education, research, and service. Historically, it is appropriate to note—without detracting from its significance—that if it had not emerged, some other social instrument would have: society was at a decision point.

The Flexner Report was to have many influences on medical education. Its major effects were: (1) to encourage the adoption of a four-year medical school curriculum; (2) to introduce laboratory teaching exercises and to improve the quality of instruction through a full-time faculty; (3) to expand clinical teaching through the introduction of the clinical clerkship; (4) to bring the medical schools into the framework of the universities; and (5) to incorporate research into the teaching program—a different pattern from the separation of research programs into institutes, common in many other countries. The four-year curriculum was widely and rapidly adopted and became the model which has prevailed in American medical education to the present. Only recently has medical education begun to experiment with this curriculum, but even now—with the exception of a few new schools—the basic departmental structure has almost never been altered.

The reorganization of medical education was facilitated by the grants of the General Education Board of the Rockefeller Foundation which distributed seventy-eight million dollars among the medical schools of twenty-four universities from 1910 to 1928. The momentum for change generated by Abraham Flexner was maintained by this grant program, for he became a member of the staff of the General Education Board following the completion of his report.

The innovative spirit which ushered in the new curriculum was described by Flexner as follows:

The proprietary medical schools of the United States just described were mainly private businesses. A few of them—Harvard and Pennsylvania, for example—were in name and in law university departments, but they lacked university standards, ideals, and facilities. At the very beginning of his Harvard presidency, Dr. Eliot began the struggle to make Harvard Medical School a genuine university department in this sense. Similar steps were subsequently taken elsewhere. The movement did not, however, gain great momentum until in the last decade of the century Johns Hopkins Medical School, a university faculty in approximately the German sense, made a success in Baltimore. The lines on which the school was developed had been previously laid down by the president and trustees and their counselors; they were distinctly enunciated when the university was opened in 1876. Even so, within the field of medicine, Johns Hopkins Medical School was a bold and at the same time a singularly naive departure. Its faculty was a group of young men whose training in England, France, and Germany made them painfully aware of the wretched conditions generally obtaining in the United States. Without asking themselves whether their plans harmonized, or did not harmonize, with our native genius, whether they were, or were not, a natural development out of existing conditions, whether on the terms proposed they could, or could not, recruit either a teaching staff or a student body, they welded in a new pattern the soundest features of French, English, and German medical education, doing, without thought of consequences, the logical, rather than the prudential, thing.[2]

The very excellence of this program, which was copied nationwide, became a potent inhibitor of further curriculum innovation in the ensuing decades.

The changes suggested by the Flexner Report could be accomplished only through the introduction of an institutional accreditation process or by licensing or certification of the practitioner. Both approaches were employed; the Association of American Medical Colleges developed a standard curriculum which was incorporated in its by-laws as a requirement for membership, and the Council on Medical Education of the American Medical Association included the standard curriculum in its statement of essentials of an approved medical school. This statement of essentials became the basis for accreditation of the medical schools. For those who have not looked upon the AMA as a crusading organization, it is appropriate to note that this was a courageous action, for many of the members of the AMA had graduated from the very schools which the accrediting process would eliminate. For almost four decades schools were rated A, B, or C as various accommodations took place, and it was not until 1949 that the last of the "unapproved" schools moved into the "approved" category and there remained no stratification among medical schools in the United States. (The schools of osteopathy have been undergoing continuing improvement also; one has recently become an accredited school of medicine.)

As part of the process of accommodation, accreditation was accorded some schools with sufficient resources to meet standards even without the acquisition of a university affiliation. Ten such schools, in existence today, graduate approximately 10 percent of the physicians in the United States. One may speculate that, if efforts had been made to keep many more such schools in existence (since universities seemed reluctant to take on the responsibility), the production of practitioners might have been markedly greater over the next several decades and the history of medical care might have been quite different. This point is important to contemplate, for there is a generally unanimous—and somewhat uncritical—attribution of only good consequences to the impact of the Flexner Report.

Approximately one third of the medical schools closed in the decade following the Flexner Report. Although a trend toward a reduction in the number of medical school graduates preceded the publication of the report, it probably accelerated the trend. Thus by 1919 there were about half the number of graduates as in 1900 (figure 1); it was not until after World War II that the number of medical school graduates returned to the level of 1900. The decline in the number of graduates was paralleled by a reduction in the number of physicians (figure 2).

The second regulatory effect was through licensure for practice, a responsibility of the individual states. Although these responsibilities overlapped with those of accreditation (the close collaboration of the accrediting agency, the Council on Medical Education of the AMA, and the state licensing boards is perhaps best symbolized in their joint annual meeting), there

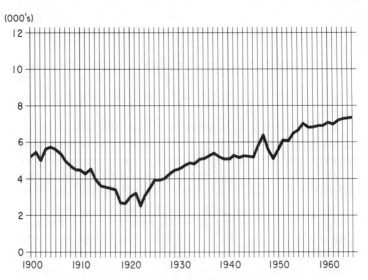

Fig. 1. Graduates of medical schools, 1900–1965.
SOURCE: Adapted from U.S. Bureau of the Census, *Historical Statistics of the United States: Colonial Times to 1957* (Washington, D. C., 1960), p. 34, and U.S. Bureau of the Census, *Statistical Abstracts of the United States:* vol. 1967 (Washington, D. C., 1967), p. 68.

were exceptions which formed the basis for the continued existence of the nonaccredited schools. As long as a student had the prospect of attaining licensure in even one state, such schools could continue to recruit students. The licensing responsibilities of the states served to introduce an additional inhibiting effect on curriculum innovation; the statutes of the various states (patterned after the recommendations of the Association of American Medical Colleges and the American Medical Association) often prescribed the curriculum in considerable detail —even to minimum hours of instruction in individual subjects. In a recent editorial comment on proposed curriculum changes at the Harvard Medical School, the editors of *The New England Journal of Medicine* noted that change may be made difficult by licensing requirements.[3]

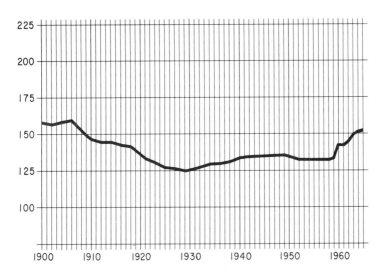

Fig. 2. Physicians (per 100,000 population), 1900–1965.
SOURCE: Adapted from U.S. Bureau of the Census, *Historical Statistics of the United States: Colonial Times to 1957* (Washington, D.C., 1960), p. 34, and U.S. Bureau of the Census. *Statistical Abstracts of the United States:* vols. 1958–1967 (Washington, D.C.).

The AMA and Public Policy

During the second decade of this century, while reductions in the numbers of medical students and physicians were under way, major issues concerning medical care and its financing were occupying the profession. As Freymann has so lucidly recorded, the matter of health insurance was debated fully within organized medicine.[4] A report of the AMA Committee on Social Insurance in 1917 suggested that the profession cooperate in efforts to formulate insurance laws dealing with all matters of medical aid. The report was commended to the state societies in the interest of the health of the people. This attitude was in marked contrast to the later opposition to all forms of health insurance.[5]

With the exception of programs on more scientific issues like quackery, drug testing, and the "seal of acceptance" program for foods and drugs (which was discontinued in the mid-1950's), the 1917 report was probably the last flexible, nondoctrinaire action taken on a matter of public policy by the AMA over the next several decades. For by 1920 the die was cast; with a limited number of physicians being educated and with the complexity of education and medical care increasing, the AMA began to reflect more and more what were believed to be the interests of its members. This trend was undoubtedly augmented by the depression of the thirties during which time many physicians were not fully employed and suffered the same severe economic problems as the rest of the population. That this was a matter of underutilization and not of lack of medical need was made abundantly evident in the National Health Survey of 1935–36.[6]

In my opinion, the impact of the depression years on the considerable limitation of the growth of medical education has not received adequate emphasis. The several years of economic privation which many physicians faced during this period (often followed by several years of limited income in military service during World War II) are still vivid in the minds of many who occupy positions of leadership even today. It may be difficult—if not impossible—to consider any significant expansion while this generation of physicians occupies leadership, although recently the Board of Trustees of the AMA has taken a public position advocating the education of more physicians.[7] Conversely, it is difficult for young physicians today to imagine large numbers of physicians relatively idle because patients were unable to afford private medical care (one-third of the physicians had incomes below $5,000 per year during the depression). These same influences (low income during the depression and limited income during military service in World War II—fifteen years of what should be the most productive years of professional persons) may also account in part for the rigid political conservatism of medical leadership during the two decades following World War II. There are signs that physicians educated after World War II, who have known only an affluent period, will be more flexible, more pragmatic, and less doctrinaire in their attitudes toward public policy and social change.

Freymann noted that until the early 1920's the leadership of the AMA was made up predominantly of the scientific and educational leadership in medicine, and suggested that a reorientation of its policies would require a return of these figures to the political structure of the AMA.[4] But this approach neglects the rich socio-historical forces which drew them away, and it overlooks the possibility that in the expression of professional opinion concerning public policy a multilithic—rather than a monolithic—approach might be preferable. Certainly American physicians have not benefited unconditionally from the popular impression that on all matters they have a monolithic stand which is expressed by the AMA. A multiplicity of organizations, the "colleges" and "academies" of specialists, each with its orientation toward public policy emerged. In many ways these organizations became more representative of the views of physicians. Because of their more limited resources, their policies were not given the wide public exposure accorded the AMA's positions.

Several factors tended to set the scientific and professional leadership off in a different direction from the political leadership (however, this should not be oversimplified; the scientific leadership developed a "politics" of its own). The professionalization of medical education consumed the scientific leaders more and more. It was no longer possible to give a series of lectures and thereby discharge one's obligations to students. Laboratory and clinical instruction became more and more demanding. A corollary was the growth of research, stimulated considerably by the theoretical and methodological advances in the sciences. As clinical investigation became more structured and complex, a corps of full-time clinical investigators developed, with an allegiance to their scientific disciplines in the university as well as to their clinical disciplines in the community.

Concomitant with the growth of scientific knowledge and clinical investigation was the emergence of specialization. Apparently, it was not the dislike of organizational tasks that kept the scientific leaders in the profession from working within the AMA. They went about forming their "academies" and "colleges" with considerable energy and enthusiasm from the 1920's on, in spite of the fact that the "sections" of the AMA might have served this purpose. (These sections still exist within the AMA but continue to attract little interest; their fate is a matter for recurrent debate within AMA councils.)

The medical schools were beginning to manifest some organizational autonomy. The Association of American Medical Colleges, an organization made up of institutional members of the medical schools, although organized in 1876, had served as little more than a clearing house for information among the medical schools. Early in this century it was drawn into the process of accreditation of medical schools in collaboration with the Council on Medical Education of the AMA. The AAMC rarely took a position on public policy in the years between the World Wars. Following World War II it became much more active.

The large organizational structure of the AMA, although intended to assure a democratic process, apparently did not provide congenial auspices for the growth of these new professional organizations. The gradual preoccupation of the AMA with political issues tended to blunt concern for professional issues; only secondarily were the new groups concerned with matters of public policy. Recently, as these organizations have grown in size and age, they have begun to assume the cumbersome, more bureaucratic structure of the AMA. (An interesting general study of the process of bureaucratization of professional organizations has been presented by Gilb.[8])

For the individual physician the climb up the organizational ladder in the AMA—from the county through the district and state societies, the House of Delegates, and perhaps finally to the Board of Trustees—became more and more arduous and time consuming. This sequence resulted in a Board of Trustees whose members have generally been above sixty years of age and who have reached this position because of their conservative views, a situation which has probably contributed to the adoption of policies oriented to the past or to the status quo. A greater and greater AMA preoccupation with political issues has caused many, in recent years, to propose that it give up any efforts at professional educational activities. At the level of the county medical societies the low attendance at meetings became a chronic concern of the officers of the Association.

The decade of the twenties and the "quest for normalcy" after World War I was characterized by little social ferment—and medicine was no exception. There was little significant public or professional pressure for change, although the costs of medical care aroused sufficient concern to result in the establishment in 1927 of a Committee on the Costs of Medical Care, which was supported by the contributions of several foundations and agencies. The Committee was headed by Ray Lyman Wilbur, M.D., and counted among its members distinguished physicians and medical economists Michael M. Davis, I. S. Falk, Nathan Sinai, and many others who continued to serve as leading spokesmen for constructive change over the next several decades. Adequate recognition was never accorded the staff and members of the Committee for the comprehensiveness of their work and the resourcefulness of their recommendations; these recommendations anticipated virtually all the changes that developed in later decades in health services and financing. Indeed its recommendations, resulting from the twenty-six volume report, have not yet been attained fully, as a review of them will show:

12

Recommendation 1.—The Committee recommends that medical service, both preventive and therapeutic, should be furnished largely by organized groups of physicians, dentists, nurses, pharmacists, and other associated personnel. Such groups should be organized, preferably around a hospital, for rendering complete home, office, and hospital care. The form of organization should encourage the maintenance of high standards and the development or preservation of a personal relation between patient and physician.

1A. Community Medical Centers. The Committee's most fundamental specific proposal is the development of suitable hospitals into comprehensive community medical centers, with branches and medical stations where needed, in which the medical professions and the public participate in the provision of, and the payment for, all health and medical care, with the professional aspects of the service under the control of professional personnel. Existing hospitals may become community medical centers by (1) including general practitioners as well as specialists on their staffs and providing office space for these practitioners, (2) organizing medical, dental and nursing staffs as a group complying with the essentials of satisfactory medical service set forth in Chapter II, and (3) accepting responsibility for furnishing complete medical service for the local population or for some section thereof. This need not interfere with the reception of other patients. Group clinics may become medical centers through the provision of home service, the addition of hospital facilities or affiliation with an existing hospital, and the formation of a representative community board to counsel and advise the clinic. Industrial and university medical services may expand into medical centers by similar procedures. The services of community medical centers must be coordinated with some plan of group payment. The functions of a community medical center will probably include various clinical, therapeutic, and preventive services which are now often provided by official health agencies. This fact should not, however, impair to any degree the authority, responsibility, or administrative functions of the health department.

Recommendation 2.—The Committee recommends the extension of all basic public health services—whether provided by governmental or non-governmental agencies—so that they will be available to the entire population according to its needs. Primarily this extension requires increased financial support for official health departments and full-time trained health officers and members of their staffs whose tenure is dependent only upon professional and administrative competence.

Recommendation 3.—The Committee recommends that the costs of medical care be placed on a group payment basis, through the use of insurance, through the use of taxation, or through the use of both these methods. This is not meant to preclude the continuation of medical service provided on an individual fee basis for those who prefer the present method. Cash benefits, i.e., compensation for wage-loss due to illness, if and when provided, should be separate and distinct from medical services.

Recommendation 4.—The Committee recommends that the study, evaluation, and coordination of medical service be considered important functions for every state and local community, that agencies be formed to exercise these functions, and that the coordination of rural with urban services receive special attention.

Recommendation 5.—The Committee makes the following recommendations in the field of professional education: (A) That the training of physicians give increasing emphasis to the teaching of health and the prevention of disease; that more effective efforts be made to provide trained health officers; that the social aspects of medical practice be given greater attention; that specialties be restricted to those specially qualified; and that postgraduate educational opportunities be increased; (B) that dental students be given a broader educational background; (C) that pharmaceutical education place more stress on the pharmacist's responsibilities and opportunities for public service; (D) that nursing education be thoroughly remoulded to provide well-educated and well-qualified registered nurses; (E) that less thoroughly trained but competent nursing aides or attendants be provided; (F) that adequate training for nurse-midwives be provided; and (G) that opportunities be offered for the systematic training of hospital and clinical administrators.[9]

It is difficult in retrospect to comprehend the relative neglect of the report of this committee. The depression years and the concomitant preoccupation with economic survival—national and individual—at the time of the report in 1932 probably resulted in assigning a relatively low priority to medical care. Consumers had not yet developed an organized concern for health services, and the makers of public policy (congressmen and state legislators) had not yet appreciated the latent interest of the people in financing more and better medical care.

The health services within the government were concentrated in the United States Public Health Service (USPHS) which originated through a Congressional Act of 1798 and was charged with the responsibility for medical service to sick and disabled seamen (out of which developed the Marine Hospitals). This program was financed by monthly contributions of twenty cents deducted from each seaman's wage and was the first compulsory sickness insurance plan in the United States. The contributory feature was later eliminated and costs were paid from general taxation. The USPHS gradually developed a broader public health responsibility and relationships with state and local health departments. It provided services for specific federal programs, such as the Indian Bureau of the Department of Interior. It developed a sophistication in the collection of health statistics and conducted various studies which highlighted significant health problems of the nation from time to time, for example, the National Health Survey of 1935–36. Its responsibilities for fostering health research increased, and it became the major agency in the nation financing these programs.[10] But it had little tradition in the broader area of medical care and its delivery.

In response to the Flexner Report, the medical schools were improving and expanding their teaching and research facilities. Aside from the provision of some services for the low income population through teaching hospitals and clinics, they did not engage in exploratory programs in delivering medical care. The schools of public health, few in number, were oriented toward the tradition of teaching epidemiology and public health administration with relatively little emphasis on medical care patterns. This orientation reflected the general concern of public health officials with problems of sanitary engineering and infectious disease control. Some recognition of the need for additional health services was evident in the Social Security Act of 1936. Significantly, these first major medical care programs— which authorized grants to the states for maternal and child health and crippled children's programs—were placed in the Children's Bureau and not the USPHS. These programs provided for a variety of administrative alternatives in their implementation and were quite effective in developing high standards of care.

The same trend was apparent in 1950 when the Social Security amendment for vendor (fee for service) payments under Public Assistance was enacted; responsibility was placed in the Welfare Administration and the state and local Welfare— rather than Health—Departments.

To repeat, the recommendations of the Committee on the Costs of Medical Care found few advocates, but strong and vocal antagonists. The across-the-board refusal of the AMA to consider any change, including hospitalization insurance, which came to be rather commonplace within the next decades, has been described by historians of this period. In retrospect it is striking that the AMA's strongest argument—that the health of the American people was the best in the world because of its system of medical care—was received with so much credulity. It should be said here that health statistics measure so many factors that it becomes very difficult to claim a distinctly better state for one developed nation over another. But most significantly the very improvements in health for which the AMA took credit had little to do with fee-for-service practice of medicine. Thus infant mortality probably was reduced as much or more as a consequence of the introduction of pasteurization of milk in 1913, the advent of public health practices, immunization for several infectious diseases, and improved standards of living, than as a result of the work of the individual practitioner.

Recognition of the continuing need for a vigorous attack on the nation's health problems by physicians was reflected in the organization of a study of physicians' opinions by the American Foundation Studies in Government. Its report of 1937, *American Medicine: Expert Testimony Out of Court,* was based on 5,000 communications from approximately 2,100 physicians and formed a rich summary of currents and crosscurrents in American medicine.[11]

The intransigence of the AMA and its lack of response to this report led to the organization of a Committee of Physicians, popularly known as the "Committee of 430" because of the number of distinguished physicians who initially sponsored the statement of principles and proposals. The explanatory statement of the Committee and its principles and proposals were as follows:

A large number of medical men believe that the report of the American Foundation Studies in Government, entitled American Medicine: Expert Testimony Out of Court deserves the thoughtful attention of physicians.

As a contribution to the discussion of the subject of medical care in the United States, this self-appointed group of medical men, finding themselves in agreement, have formulated certain principles and proposals anent such care. These physicians, who have been trying to purvey medical care for many years, speak only for themselves and not for the Foundation or for any other organization. They hope that these principles and proposals may suggest the lines along which effort may be made by voluntary, local, state and federal agencies to improve medical care.

It is recognized that the medical profession is only one of several groups to which "medical care" is of vital concern. Close cooperation between physicians, economists and sociologists is essential. Nevertheless the medical profession should initiate any proposed changes because physicians are the experts upon whom communities must depend. Unless the medical profession is ready to cooperate with these other groups, physicians cannot expect to play successfully the part which they should play, nor can they expect to enlist the sympathetic understanding of legislative bodies.

It seems to us probable that certain alterations in our present system of preventing illness and providing medical care may become necessary; indeed, certain changes have already occurred. Medical knowledge is increasing rapidly and is becoming more complex. Changes in economic and social conditions are taking place at home and abroad. Medicine must be mobile and not static if medical men are to act as the expert advisers of those who convert public opinion into action.

The conviction is general that action should be taken only upon the basis of demonstrated need and as experience accumulates to indicate that such action is likely to attain its ends in a nation comprising forty-eight states in which climatic, economic and social conditions vary greatly.

Principles

1. That the health of the people is a direct concern of the government.
2. That a national public health policy directed toward all groups of population should be formulated.
3. That the problem of economic need and the problem of providing adequate medical care are not identical and may require different approaches for their solution.
4. That in the provision of adequate medical care for the population four agencies are concerned: voluntary agencies, local, state and federal governments.

Proposals

1. That the first necessary step toward the realization of the above principles is to minimize the risk of illness by prevention.

18

2. That an immediate problem is provision of adequate medical care for the medically indigent, the cost to be met from public funds (local and/or state and/or federal).
3. That public funds should be made available for the support of medical education and for studies, investigations and procedures for raising the standards of medical practice. If this is not provided for, the provision of adequate medical care may prove impossible.
4. That public funds should be available for medical research as essential for high standards of practice in both preventive and curative medicine.
5. That public funds should be made available to hospitals that render service to the medically indigent and for laboratory and diagnostic and consultative services.
6. That in allocation of public funds existing private institutions should be utilized to the largest possible extent and that they may receive support so long as their service is in consonance with the above principles.
7. That public health services, federal, state and local, should be extended by evolutionary process.
8. That the investigation and planning of the measures proposed and their ultimate direction should be assigned to experts.
9. That the adequate administration and supervision of the health functions of the government, as implied in the above proposals, necessitates in our opinion a functional consolidation of all federal health and medical activities, preferably under a separate department.

The subscribers to the above principles and proposals hold the view that health insurance alone does not offer a satisfactory solution on the basis of the principles and proposals enunciated above.[12]

The opposition of the AMA was prompt. To quote an editorial on the formation of the Committee from the *Journal of the American Medical Association:*

It should not be necessary to point out again in THE JOURNAL the danger of federal subsidies for medical schools and the hazard of turning over to the federal government the control and standardization of medical schools. Such subsidies may easily involve determination of the curriculum and administration of service through the medical schools which would quite certainly interfere with the advancement of medical education and medical science and put the government right into the practice of medicine. Already, in some foreign countries, the government controls the number of medical students and the nature of medical education. American medicine wants no such system. Our government has already voted $750,000 a year for the control of cancer and suggestions have been offered that similar appropriations be made for the study of infantile paralysis, syphilis and other diseases. The danger of putting the government in the dominant position in relation to medical research is apparent.

Still more serious is the fifth proposal, to the effect that the government subsidize private hospitals in relationship to their laboratory, diagnostic and consultative services. The nonprofit voluntary hospital is the pride of American philanthropy and a major factor in maintaining a high quality of medical service. The tender of governmental funds to such institutions for the care of an ill defined group called the medically indigent appeals to the unthinking physicians who have endorsed these principles and proposals. Yet such an arrangement would put the hospitals promptly into the practice of medicine . . .

Obviously some of these men must have signed merely after seeing the names of those who signed previously and because it looked like a "good" list. There appear also the names of some members of the House of Delegates which voted against some of the very propositions which these members here support. Most conspicuous on the list are the names of those deans and heads of departments in medical schools who may have signed because they saw a possibility of getting government money for clinics and dispensaries.

Such careless participation in propaganda as has here occurred is lamentable, to say the least. Certainly the unthinking endorsers of the American Foundation's principles and proposals owe to the medical profession some prompt disclaimers.[13]

The vitriolic nature of the attacks on the Committee reflected the increasingly doctrinaire position which was evolving in the

AMA, and which was responsible for some harassment of members of the Committee. These attacks, in addition to a preoccupation with the military mobilization, led to the gradual disappearance of this courageous group. The lack of a staff and organizational base and the very informality of the manner in which the Committee was organized probably contributed to its demise. But its members pointed the way toward changes that were to develop following World War II.

The Specialization of Medical Manpower

During the twenties, and even more during the thirties, it became increasingly apparent that advances in the medical sciences and in technology necessitated training beyond the four years of medical school. The one or two years of internship, with occasional exceptions in some academic institutions, was general training and did not provide the specialized training which was becoming recognized as a requisite for improving the quality of care. At the time the internship was a requirement for licensure, although its statutory specifications varied from state to state. Specialized (or "straight") internships were offered in a few medical centers—mainly in the East—before World War II and the number rapidly increased following the war, but it was not until the early 1960's that Illinois and Pennsylvania revised their statutes to permit the licensure of a candidate who had served a straight internship.

The accrediting agency for the internship was the Council on Medical Education and Hospitals of the AMA. The accrediting process was quite independent of the medical schools. Since the advantages of interns for the hospital were many, there were great pressures to approve hospitals for internship training. And since the internship grew up during a period when the educational requirements for a desirable program were not complex, many hospitals were accredited for internship training which could not in later years mount the educational program thought to be essential for a good internship. This process resulted in the ultimate listing of more than twice the number of internship positions than there were medical school graduates as applicants, for once a hospital had gained approval, it became very difficult to remove it from the accredited list. The system worked in such a way that an intense competition for applicants gradually developed among the hospitals.

As the scientific and professional leaders in medicine moved toward the establishment of their specialty organizations—the "academies" and "colleges"—the matter of specialty training began to concern them more and more. (The role of the academies, as contrasted to the universities, as forces for learning and scholarship is not a new one in this century. The medical historian, Henry Sigerist, deals with their role in the seventeenth, eighteenth, and nineteenth centuries and their impact on university education. [14]) Gradually nineteen boards in the medical specialties were established during the thirties, coordinated by an Advisory Board for the medical specialties. Although each specialty board had autonomous corporate status, a pattern of representation by the specialty societies, the academic societies in each specialty, and the specialty section of the AMA was rather common to each of the boards. Hospitals had a large stake in having residents as well as interns and relatively large numbers of residency positions were approved for the training of specialists. Again, as in the internship, the educational and training needs grew to a complexity which many hospitals could not meet. A decade later, in the late forties, the situation resulted in intense competition for applicants on the basis of noneducational benefits (such as higher salaries and living quarters) which could be provided more readily than the educational program. It should be noted that interns and residents of the pre-World War II period were paid little or nothing beyond room and board on the basis that they were receiving an educational experience, although they were more than eight years beyond high school. One wonders whether this pattern of low income for such a highly educated group could have developed if residency programs had not been initiated mainly during the depression years.

Just as the Flexner Report established an enduring pattern for the organization of the medical school, so the specialty boards established an enduring pattern in the twenties and thirties for the training of specialists. Although university medical centers provide a considerable proportion of the residency training programs, the responsibility for accreditation resides mainly outside the universities. Also the numbers of positions approved for training are based on the capacity of the hospitals to provide training opportunities; the matter of the needs of the nation for specialists of various kinds does not tend to enter into the accreditation process. There have been efforts from time to time to recruit trainees for specialties in which there are critical shortages, with the recruitment incentives largely in the form of increased stipends. The relatively chaotic nature of the post-medical school training programs and the fact that they represent a time investment by the trainee equal to his medical student days stimulated the Board of Trustees of the AMA to appoint a Citizens' Commission on Graduate Medical Education in 1963—with the hope that it would do for postgraduate education what the Flexner Report did for the medical school. This commission rendered its report in 1966 (The Millis Report).[15]

By World War II the trend toward specialization was well under way—never to be reversed. The military services had not yet accommodated to this shift and in the early days of the war held to the notion that every physician was to be interchangeable with another. But inevitably the military services had to recognize the waste of skill which was taking place under this system, and there was increasing awareness that proper development of specialists meant better medical care, which could not be denied to patients as more specialists entered military service. Thus the military occupational specialty designation came to include the medical specialties, and by the end of the war there were significant efforts to match the specialist with an appropriate assignment.

The period of military service probably catalyzed the trend toward specialization. Many physicians had an opportunity for more intimate contact with specialists. Indeed, following the war there developed a steady flow of physicians from general practice into specialty training in spite of exhortations to young physicians to enter general practice because of the need. Also, although many physicians experienced the frustrations of working within the large scale bureaucracy of the military establishment and vowed they would return only to fee-for-service solo practice, many also became more aware of some of the advantages of group practice or institutional work of some kind. Although a trend away from individual practice had begun prior to World War II, it continued steadily after the War, from 86 percent in individual practice in 1931 to 63 percent in 1962.

It is interesting to speculate when this trend might begin to manifest itself in the power structure (and therefore public policy formation) of the AMA. Although one may question why more diversification has not as yet manifested itself within the AMA as a result of the trend, it is apparent that physicians in group or institutional programs feel their interests are in general reflected by their institutional affiliation (universities, public health departments, the Veteran's Administration, and other federal agencies) or by the organizations which support these interests (such as the Association of American Medical Colleges, academic professional societies, the American Public Health Association, the Group Health Association of America). However, many individual practitioners still see the AMA as the major—and often sole—guardian of their interests and therefore work hard to make it so. (A lucid account of the problems of this group has been presented by Somers.[16]) But for reasons already mentioned, some physicians find the climb through the AMA organization too tedious and cumbersome to pursue. The analyst of social organizations may speculate that, when the critical mass of fee-for-service practitioners declines to a certain level (perhaps 50 percent), the policy orientation of the AMA may undergo a decided shift.

By 1940 the pattern of medical education had become stabilized in contrast to the chaotic conditions prior to the Flexner Report. The trend toward specialization was well under way and the structure of specialty training programs had become well established. Medical and other health professional organizations grew in numbers and strength. Although the passage of the Social Security Act had some implications for health programs, there was little additional ferment. Was this a calm before the storm of change which was evolving?

2   The Scientific Revolution and the Academic

Establishment (1940–1960)

Research, Government, and the University

By the end of World War II the incorporation of scientific advances into medical practice was occurring at a rapid pace. The introduction of antibacterial drugs, the newer knowledge of the action of hormones, the replacement of blood, plasma, and fluids which had become common during the war, and the increasing complexity and effectiveness of surgery heightened general expectations for the preservation and lengthening of life. The seemingly infinite productive capacity of the nation during the war, enhanced by the brilliant success of scientists in the application of their knowledge of atomic energy through the Manhattan Project, fortified the expectation that no result was unattainable if the resources were adequate. The limitations of this point of view are dealt with comprehensively in a report of a conference on "Research in the Service of Man" in which Dr. Alvin Weinberg, Director of the Oak Ridge National Laboratory, differentiates basic and applied approaches—or feasibility and nonfeasibility—as follows:

there is a difference between the physical and biological sciences with respect to the degree to which their underlying scientific structure can be efficiently mobilized for achieving practical goals. The physical sciences and engineering, though they may have started independently . . . have now been so intertwined and integrated, and the physical sciences themselves are so advanced, that given an applied goal in engineering, there is often nothing but money that stands in the way of achieving the goal,

27

provided basic science has shown this goal to be achievable. I can't stress too strongly the importance of this latter proviso. Thus, applications in the physical sciences fall into two great categories; those projects whose basic feasibility has been demonstrated and those equally desirable projects whose feasibility is yet to be demonstrated . . . The bulk of biomedical research is in the pre-feasibility stage, and therefore, the underlying basic research must be done broadly. Since most of our knowledge is in the pre-feasibility stage, the vital link between basic and applied biomedical research is much more haphazard and unpredictable than I suspect our President would like it to be . . . I think it is fair to say that most basic molecular biologists would work directly on a cure for cancer rather than on what they are now doing, if only they knew how to make real progress. We don't cure cancer because we don't want to, but rather because we don't know how to cure it.[1]

The medical schools as the major medical research institu-. tions of the country were receptive to the challenge. The long period of institutionalizing the educational program in the prewar years—and particularly the depression years—did not permit much institutional growth. But by now theoretical and methodological advances in the sciences stimulated the pressures for research expansion. The universities, bursting at the seams attempting to accommodate the influx of returning veterans, seemed to be in no position to provide the resources for these efforts. And the foundations, traditionally a major source of support for medical research during the prewar period, found their resources increasingly inadequate in the face of growing requests.

Since support for medical research efforts was not so controversial as support for medical care, it did not seem politically hazardous to propose that federal appropriations would be a logical source of support. (An extremely skilful and effective combined citizen, scientist, and legislator force developed which catalyzed the trend toward federal funding. The activities of this group have been described by Drew.[2]) Another possible source might have been state funds—especially for the state-sponsored medical schools. Actually some support did come directly from state university budgets, but the states were encountering increasing fiscal difficulties because of the high priorities for highways, schools, and support of the state-operated health and welfare institutions. Also the private universities might have been at a considerable disadvantage under this arrangement, and since, especially in the East, they had a tradition of political as well as academic strength, this channel was not pursued in a major way. (These comments are of course interpretative since a clear delineation of, or struggle over, these alternatives never took place.)

The governmental agency which seemed the most logical haven for a research-funding program was the Public Health Service of the then Federal Security Agency, which later was to be incorporated into the new Department of Health, Education and Welfare. The specific subdivision through which appropriations and expenditures were to be made was the National Institutes of Health (NIH), made up of a group of individual institutes that evolved pragmatically out of concerns with specific organs (the National Heart Institute), diseases (the National Cancer Institute), or both (the National Institute of Neurological Diseases and Blindness). It was not until 1962 that institutes concerned with processes rather than organs or diseases were established (the National Institute of Child Health and Human Development, and the National Institute on the General Medical Sciences). As for the AMA, aside from occasional expressions of concern over the size of expenditures and possible federal control of research, it did not strongly oppose this development, probably because it was becoming increasingly involved in campaigns to oppose legislative proposals for health insurance which were supported by President Truman and various congressional leaders.

The almost universal acceptance of the research effort resulted in its becoming the fastest growing component of all national health expenditures, which increased from $12.9 bil-

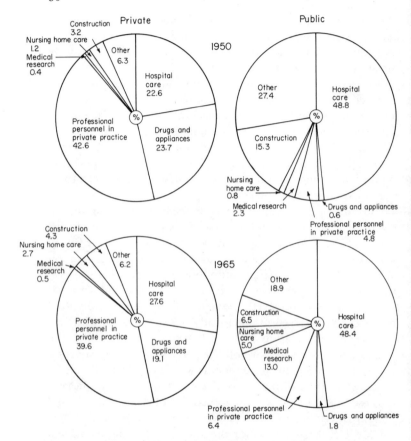

Fig. 3. Distribution (percent) of private and public expenditures, by object of expenditure, 1950 and 1965. "Other" private expenditures include those for the net cost of health insurance, private voluntary health agencies, and industrial in-plant health services. "Other" public expenditures include those for government public health activities; medical activities in federal units other than hospitals, and school health services. Total expenditures for 1950: private, $9.3 billion; public, $3.6 billion; for 1965: private, $30.5 billion; public, $10.2 billion.
Source: R. Hanft, "National Health Expenditures, 1950–65," *Social Security Bulletin 30*:3 (February 1967).

lion in 1950 to $40.7 billion in 1965. During this same period research expenditures increased from $117 million to $1.5 billion. Less than 1 percent of the health expenditures in 1950, in 1965 it constituted 3.7 percent. Most of this increase was from the federal government, since its support for health research rose from $79 million to $1.3 billion during these years (figure 3).[3]

These expenditures were implemented through an interesting scientific-political power structure. In order to assure scientific competence in the awarding of grants, the staff of NIH developed a review process; a study section made up of nongovernmental scientists drawn mainly from the universities and an advisory council made up of professional persons and a few citizens-at-large were provided for each institute. This arrangement served as a jury system to share the responsibility for judgments while at the same time providing a bicameral process of review (study sections–advisory councils) and insurance against governmental bureaucratic or political controls over the expenditures, and it provided Congress with the assurance that the research dollars were being spent on the advice of our best scientist-citizens. Since the foundations and voluntary health agencies making research grants obtained consultation from the same pool of professional persons, their programs were in many respects similar, but inasmuch as the federal funds were much larger, foundations and voluntary health agencies found it increasingly difficult to find innovative programs to support that were not eligible for federal grant support.

This policy- and decision-making process, along with the influx of dollars, was having an interesting impact on the medical schools and their universities.* The rapid growth in faculty and physical plant was mainly by accretion rather than by any institutional reorganization, and the once primary mission of teaching medical students became diluted by the more than ten-

* These developments have been dealt with in detail in a number of publications of the proceedings of "Institutes" of the AAMC [4,5,6] and such volumes as Kerr's *Multiversity* [7] and Perkins' *The University in Transition*,[8] and the "News and Comment" section of *Science* of the past several years.

fold increase in research expenditures. The relative decline of interest in teaching in favor of research was shared with the rest of the university and continues as a major problem for resolution in the modern university.[9] The problems of growth, common to all medical schools, varied in magnitude among them, for those schools with a longer tradition of research were in a more favorable position to attract research grants, with the result that the rich got richer while the traditionally poor institutions experienced a much slower expansion.

With the influx of research grants and personnel the role of the university and medical school administration became increasingly ambiguous in determining the rate and nature of the growth. During the prewar period the university administration determined the allocation of space and funds, but now the funds were attracted to the universities predominantly through the individual faculty members. And faculty members, as individual entrepreneurs saw mainly the advantages which their research grants brought to the universities. The administrators in the main saw all the same advantages at first, but later they began to struggle with the institutional stresses brought on by the influx of money and staff. Administrators were faced with the necessity of providing institutional support in the form of space (including matching funds for construction) and supporting services.

The somewhat differing perspectives of research worker and administrator are perhaps best illustrated by the attitudes concerning the adequacy of the provision for overhead costs as part of NIH research grants. This is a provision which was increased from 15 to 20 percent of the grant in recent years to help compensate the university for the overhead involved (often referred to as indirect costs) in the operation of the grant (for example, maintenance, heat, light, and telephones). The research worker generally felt the amount was adequate; the administrator, especially if his institution receives many grants, felt that it was inadequate. Congress and the Bureau of the Budget, interested in supporting both groups while protecting the taxpayer, worry

about arriving at a just figure and have substituted a plan for
cost-sharing by the university, in which the university is required to make a contribution of 5 percent of the total cost to
the support of research and is paid for the indirect costs as cal-
culated by periodic audits. This has resulted gradually in the
development of considerable administrative complexity on the
part of the government and the universities. In the program for
the support of construction for research facilities, Congress has
specified the equal sharing of costs by the institution and the
federal government (except for facilities for mental retardation
for which the government share is 75 percent). Although this
was a welcome basis in the early days of the program, institutions are finding it more and more difficult to provide their
share of the matching funds. The result is increasing pressure
for the federal government to provide a much higher percentage
—or all—of the construction funds.

The matter of arriving at overhead costs by cost accounting
procedures may seem simple to the outsider, but when one re-
calls that research is going on in the same institution with education and patient care (and often involves patient care), some
idea of the complexity of the problem may be appreciated. In
spite of this, persistent and creative efforts to determine costs
have gone on in recent years.[9, 10, 11]

The faculty members, through their representation on policy
making committees, determine the nature of the grants and the
institutional ground rules. At any one time over 600 biomedical
scientists are on various NIH study sections and councils; the
membership is rotating and a large number have participated
in this process. The influence of these groups is particularly potent, because the grant funds are distributed mainly on the basis
of project grant applications by individual investigators.

The process of reviewing project grant applications by the
study sections has gradually become a very large scale administrative operation. Because of the time necessary for the reading
and study of applications, the time spent at study section meetings, and the time required for site visits (visiting the applicant

investigators and institutions) an elaborate extramural establishment has grown up. Amusing, but not entirely facetious, anecdotes illustrate the problems: the medical school faculty that was having difficulty in mustering a quorum for a meeting of senior faculty members because of these outside commitments; or the comments of some deans that "full-time faculty" now means full time away from home; or "the dean who on one day counted 33 site visitors on his campus." [12] In connection with construction grants, it has become common to have site visits by two or three different study sections and their staffs. For medical school administrators this seems to have been the straw that broke the camel's back, for they have addressed a strong resolution to the Secretary of HEW suggesting relief from this administrative complexity.[13]

Because of the large scale complexity of administering the present research program through the same mechanism that was developed when it was a small program, revisions have been suggested from time to time. The most common proposal is for a program of institutional grants which would put the controls for the distribution of funds back where they were prior to World War II—in the hands of the university. The university faculty members—in their capacities as advisors in the study sections and advisory councils—have generally resisted this possibility. Obviously institutional grants to the universities necessitate policy decisions that are difficult to make. Should disproportionately larger amounts go to the weak institutions or to those with demonstrated capacities and greater resources? (Occasional attempts have been made to deal with this matter.[14]) As the pressures for some institutional support grew, and as the rate of growth of the research funds made it increasingly difficult to expand by the project grant route, a concession was made in 1961 to provide institutional research grants. And, as though not to disturb the balance in the research establishment, the awards to institutions were based on a percentage of their research grant support for the previous year. Thus the rich remained richer.

This extramural establishment, with its divided loyalties, had a number of interesting effects on medical education. Although the loyalties were divided between the granting agency and the university, the greater loyalty tended toward the granting agency, which in many instances was the source of salaries as well as research budgets. The increasing extramural support— once called "soft money" by the universities, a term which has lost much of its meaning due to the prolonged presence of the support—created a dependence upon federal funds undreamed of two decades earlier. As a result, it has been suggested that there are no longer private universities and state universities; rather there are federal and state universities—and the latter have become very dependent upon federal funds as well. It is understandable therefore that a tendency to panic develops within the extramural (and university) establishments if there are suggestions of lagging federal support or of budget cuts for research.[15] That the highest federal officials are aware of the situation which has been created was evident in the following comment by William D. Carey,[16] Assistant Director of the Bureau of the Budget: "Government is not likely to lose sight of the hard reality that in one way or another it will have to provide for the growth and stability of the academic institutions." *

Any establishment tends to perpetuate itself and this one, accustomed to free inquiry and novelty in its own investigations, has been considerably less than innovative in relation to its institutional structure in medical centers. Indeed, although there may be some rare exceptions, it is probably fair to say that

* The first major test of the government's commitment to the growth and stability of the universities occurred in mid-1968, when reductions in the federal budget were resulting in decreases in funds for research and training programs for the first time since World War II. In June 1968, the New York Academy of Sciences sponsored an emergency meeting of 400 scientists and educators which emphasized that if federal support for science research and education were cut back heavily, the United States would suffer seriously for many years (*New York Times*, June 22, 1968, p. 9). Almost simultaneously the Association of American Universities called for a dramatic across-the-board increase in government support for all types of institutions of higher education (*New York Times*, June 24, 1968, p. 1).

there has been no major innovation or administrative creativity manifested in the administration and management of the medical centers in spite of their tremendous growth. This problem pervades the universities, not just the medical centers. Kerr, in describing the role of university administrators as mediators among the many and increasing faculty establishments with their many external loyalties, points out the great difficulty in introducing institutional change or novelty in this complex. He says of the university, "it is a pluralistic society with multiple cultures . . . The president in the multiversity is leader, educator, creator, initiator, wielder of power, pump; he is *also* office-holder, caretaker, inheritor, consensus-seeker, persuader, bottleneck. But he is mostly a mediator."

As to innovation in teaching, Jencks, in discussing higher education generally, states, "The trouble is that these faculty members rarely show anything like as much imagination and daring in their teaching as in their research." [17] He also believes that introducing change in higher education requires a coalition of a dissident minority from within the university and outside financial support for their ideas to enhance their position. Unfortunately foundations are increasingly at a disadvantage financially and because of greater public scrutiny in recent years are inclined to play it safe and not support many really novel programs. Thus, although it may have seemed unlikely some years ago, support for new developments may ultimately come from public sources. Jencks suggests that we may need a twentieth-century counterpart of the Morrill Act.

The extramural medical establishment that has evolved has had an interesting effect within medical center administration (although it has not been the only force). Since within this establishment highest prestige is accorded scientific accomplishment, there has been a subtle (and sometimes not so subtle) tendency to deprecate the significance of academic administrators such as the deans and vice-presidents for medical affairs. Indeed the perception of many in this establishment is that the dean is a fiscal agent. The search for a new dean always raises the question as to whether the faculty is interested in a weak or a strong dean—the weak one being a fiscal agent, and the strong one having some potential for academic leadership. But even the strong dean, beset by a tenfold increase in budget in a decade and operating with an organizational structure of the pre-World War II days, finds himself with an almost impossible reorganizational task. (Imagine, by analogy, an industrial organization increasing its business tenfold with the same organizational apparatus. Its survival would not seem likely.) It should also be noted that, since deans have generally been drawn from the medical school faculty, they have had little or no experience with problems of institutional management and reorganization. Except for those who have come from the field of public health, or who may have had experience in hospital administration, there is virtually nothing in the educational or experiential background of a physician to prepare him for complex administrative tasks. Since relatively few have been drawn from the field of public health to medical school deanships, it is difficult to say whether such administrative background is an advantage, but on the basis of personal observation there is some reason to believe it may be.

Medical School Administration and Leadership

Some evidence of the frustration experienced by deans is perhaps apparent in the rapid turnover in these positions. A recent report indicates that the tenure of a medical school dean averaged five and a half years in 1965 (a drop from an average of seven years in 1962).[18] This situation presents a circular problem—the shorter the tenure, the less likely the dean is to come to grips with organizational problems. Since the major economic support comes from outside the university, and since this outside support has created a considerable affluence among the faculty members, it is understandable that faculty resistance to academic or administrative change would be high. Here it should be noted that this greater affluence has helped to create a critical problem not only in the medical schools but also in the federal recruitment of biomedical scientists to administer the research programs. The growing affluence of the faculty has been stimulated in no small measure by the availability of research funds from federal sources. But faculty members, for the same reasons they deprecate the administrative posts within their institutions, are perhaps even more disdainful of extra-university administrative posts. As an extramural force with influence, they have not been vigorous recruiters for these administrative posts, nor have they been active lobbyists for more adequate salaries for administrators. Over a period of time salary levels have become relatively low, making it extremely difficult to recruit first-rate people. Thus the academic establishment, by not providing adequately for quality staffing of the research establishment (while approving higher salaries for itself through research grants), has left its flank exposed. That this has become a critical matter was evident in the communication of Dr. James Shannon, Director of the National Institutes of Health, to the President.[19]

Partly because of the indifference of faculty and partly because of the growing preoccupation with research and its institutional complexity, it was not until 1952 that a medical school introduced any major curriculum revision. Western Reserve Medical School was the first to attempt revision and the first to organize the teaching program around committees of the faculty based on the functional objectives of learning rather than the traditional disciplinary (departmental) structure of the medical school. In the latter, the program is based on the background and skill of the faculty member; the new effort was to bring the faculty's skills to bear more effectively on student needs. This was probably the first major creative contribution to medical education since the introduction of the Johns Hopkins curriculum at the turn of the century. The many curriculum modifications which have come subsequently are mainly a reordering of time or sequence of existing programs or some modification of the Western Reserve program.

The deans have an organization, the Association of American Medical Colleges, which has the potentiality for leadership in shaping national policy in the fields of health services, education, and research. This organization is made up of institutional memberships (each medical school is represented through its dean—thus accounting for the frequent reference to the organization as the "deans' club"). That it has lagged in its leadership role is evident from the following comments of John Russell, President of the John and Mary R. Markle Foundation and a long time nonmedical observer of the American medical scene:

The presidents of colleges and universities are not the only ones disturbed about their growing dependence on federal grants and the growing restrictions placed on that type of support. The deans of the medical schools are also concerned—or should be. Sometimes we wonder how deeply bothered they really are, as the deans seem to be so slow about asserting their rights and protecting the freedom of their schools. With new legislation tumbling out of Washington ever faster, and with federal support now sweeping into its arms teaching and patient care as well as the time-tested medical research program, the need for the medical schools to participate in policy formation is great. Shooting out the back window after something has passed is better than nothing. However, the schools' future freedom depends on how the new laws are written and what sort of controls will accompany them.

In the past we have discussed here and elsewhere the importance of the medical educator's (all scientists', for that matter) understanding and participating in the political process. This can be done only if some agency is organized so that it represents all of academic medicine, not just a part of it. The Association of American Medical Colleges has been mentioned as the logical agency to do this. But unfortunately (at least at this writing) the Association has made no real move to reorganize. All that has been done is to open a back window in Washington from which to take pot shots at legislation already in the works or already passed.

The inability of a group of intelligent men such as medical educators to organize for political action is discouraging to anyone interested in protecting the freedom of medical schools. Sooner or later, they will have to get together, but in the meantime the advice of political scientists, skeptical of the political ability of academicians, to the effect that "if you can't beat 'em, join 'em," makes good sense.[20]

Although there has been some attempt to consider the necessary reorganization to which Russell refers, there has been little or no consistent policy and follow-through. However, awareness of a crisis was evidenced when the Association sponsored a study under the chairmanship of the distinguished medical educator (and former Assistant to the Secretary of Health, Education and Welfare), Dr. Lowell T. Coggeshall. Other members of the Committee were Dr. William N. Hubbard (Vice-Chairman), Dean, University of Michigan Medical School; Dr. Michael DeBakey, Professor of Surgery, Baylor University College of Medicine; Dr. John E. Deitrick, Dean, Cornell University Medical College; Dr. Clark Kerr, President, University of California; Dr. George A. Perera, Professor of Medicine and Associate Dean, College of Physicians and Surgeons, Columbia University; Dr. Robert C. Berson, President, Association of American Medical Colleges (1964).

This committee interpreted its charge as follows:

The enormous expansion of medical education, research, and service, especially in the past two decades, has resulted in greater changes than have occurred during any other period in our medical history. The great and growing national concern over the health of our people requires that those responsible for medical education today and in the future turn their attentions to a question of the greatest importance and most far-reaching consequences: *Will the methods and practices currently followed in providing health personnel of all categories, together with the programs and facilities in being or planned, be adequate to meet our national needs?*

This basic question about the future development of medical education, and parallel concerns about the role that the Association of American Medical Colleges should play in the decades ahead and how the organization should develop its effectiveness, led to this study of the Association's future work.[21]

In his letter of transmittal for the report, Dr. Coggeshall makes the following observations:

During the study, surprising unanimity of concern was found among medical educators, university officials, public officials, and others about problems in the field of medical education. Few persons interviewed believe improvements needed are matters of minor adjustment. Most point to the need to take major steps to improve medical education—to enable the nation to produce more and better prepared physicians and other health personnel. There is a rather consistent pattern of thought that the quality of education is good but not fully geared to future needs. Most impressive is the repeated assertion that there is need for some organization—preferably the Association of American Medical Colleges—to assume a more aggressive and correlative role if future needs in the field of education for all health personnel are to be met.[21]

Since the publication of the report, the Association has manifested its usual timidity. Although by any standards the Coggeshall Report is a comprehensive and thoughtful document (probably the best all-around discussion of health problems facing the nation in recent years) and was received with considerable interest by the press, it was for a time virtually disregarded by the Association. Except for a few hastily called regional meetings of deans to discuss some of its implications, it remains buried insofar as the proceedings of the Association are concerned. An effort to stimulate public acknowledgement of the report by the Association and to implement its recommendations was futile. The following exchange of letters between the author and the President of the Association, Dr. Thomas Turner, is illustrative:

November 17, 1965

Thomas B. Turner, M.D., President ˒
Association of American Medical Colleges
The Johns Hopkins University
School of Medicine
725 North Wolfe Street
Baltimore, Maryland 21205

Dear Doctor Turner:

Now that the Annual Meeting of the AAMC has come and gone, I feel inclined to pass some observations and comments on to you concerning the Coggeshall Report and the Association's response to it.

Everything I say is predicated on my feeling—after careful reading—that the Coggeshall Report is a brilliant pulling together of issues facing medicine and medical education in the United States today. Even though its contents are not new to most of us, its comprehensiveness, its statesmanship, its lack of any "proprietary" taint which carries its scope far beyond the immediate confines of the affairs of the AAMC—all serve to make it a document of the first importance for the people of all the United States (I might add that I've tried it out on a few intelligent non-medical citizens who uniformly regard it as a revelation). I could go on to detail my reasons for attributing such importance to it, but I don't feel this to be necessary. It speaks for itself.

Having said this, my concern is that the Executive Council has dealt with the report all too gingerly. Rather than using it as an opportunity to establish a leadership position in the U. S. by embracing the substance of the report fully—*and publicly* —I sense a tendency to try to get complete consensus on all aspects of the report. Such efforts at "playing it safe" will, I fear, put us in a position of dragging up the rear rather than moving into the lead where we belong if we really act in the spirit of the Coggeshall Report. We have the capacity for leading; I hope we won't default as some ponderous organizations have done by playing it so safe that they are decades behind the times. I am aware also that there will always be a vocal minority,

The Scientific Revolution

but I see no reason to base our policy on a least common denominator principle.

I appreciate the efforts of the Executive Council to have a full discussion among the membership. Although I yield to no one in my commitment to democratic principles, I fear that if we wait for full discussion of issues at institutional membership meetings (as was suggested at the Philadelphia meeting) we will be paralyzed. I am suggesting that the Executive Council not become defensive, but rather lead in the fashion required by the times. If the membership doesn't agree with the Council's action, it can elect new members!

Although it is commonplace to say that health legislation is developing rapidly and that times are different, the fact is that it is so. As one who has been on the Washington scene for a few months, I see no evidence that the pace will slacken. The gap in leadership from the health professions has been sufficient to be cause for concern even among those of us who are not given to "viewing with alarm" readily . . .

> Sincerely,
> Julius B. Richmond, M.D.
> Dean, The Medical Faculty

November 24, 1965

Dr. Julius B. Richmond
Dean, The Medical Faculty
State University of New York
Upstate Medical Center
766 Irving Ave.
Syracuse, N.Y. 13210

Dear Doctor Richmond:

Thank you for your encouraging and rather inspiring letter. I share your views and feel that we should move boldly into the vacuum in leadership which exists in medical affairs today. Having said this, however, it is not easy to do, for we have a touch of bureaucratic trappings in our Executive Council to the extent that there has to be some kind of consensus before anyone can move too far ahead. Second we are poorly geared up in respect to public relations, so thàt busy people are not able to strike out as they might wish. However, I think we have made progress, and many of us are in a mood to keep pushing ahead along the lines of the Coggeshall Report.*

Sincerely yours,
Thomas B. Turner, M.D.
Dean of the Medical Faculty

c.c. Dr. Robert Berson

This relative lack of leadership on the part of the medical schools is of more than passing interest. There were many who felt that the AAMC, as an organization unfettered by ties with the AMA, might emerge as the leading force for comprehensive health-program planning for the nation at a time when the AMA was deeply enmeshed in its opposition to the growing pressures for medical care for the older population. But to note the AAMC's failure is not to explain it, and there were many factors which probably contributed; among them were the following:

(1) A long history of unresponsiveness to public issues and a resultant lack of resources with which to develop a capacity for response. Prior to World War II the professional staff of the Association consisted of one physician-director. Dependent on institutional dues, the organization had not developed any financial resources with which to take on new functions. The deans, beset by their internal problems, did not see or pursue the matter of growth of the organization until after the research growth spurt was well under way. Thus it was not until 1956 that a vigorous, imaginative director, Dr. Ward Darley, was brought into the Association's offices. But by then much of the momentum for influencing health research and education had

* The author gratefully acknowledges Dr. Thomas B. Turner's permission to reproduce this correspondence.

bypassed the Association. In spite of this, Dr. Darley (against the opposition of many who said that it could not be done) undertook the study of the costs of medical education, which for the first time made specific data available for planning. He also consolidated the internal structure of the organization by rendering more effective services on student affairs to the medical schools, and stimulated research on the characteristics of medical students and the medical schools. Under the leadership of a few deans—most notably Dr. George P. Berry of the Harvard Medical School—the Association sponsored a series of national teaching institutes which heightened interest in improving the teaching programs in the medical schools.[22] That resources for expanded efforts of the Association could become available may be assumed from the support which these efforts received from several foundations. As Mr. Russell's comments indicate, there were some observers on the sidelines hoping that this group would emerge as a nonproprietary spokesman on health affairs to the nation.[12]

(2) The inexperience of many deans in dealing with public issues and legislation. Because of the rapid turnover among deans, a significant number of them were inner-directed in mastering the affairs of their institutions and therefore required some time before they could appreciate the importance of external forces affecting their programs. A number of deans, after gaining this appreciation, had left their posts. As an example of inexperience in making judgments concerning the fate of the Association, it is interesting to look at the matter of locating the Association's offices. Its quarters, long situated in downtown Chicago, were inadequate, and it became apparent that relocation was necessary. Although there was some consideration of moving to Washington where headquarters could be close to the source of national legislation, the Association made a penny-wise and pound-foolish decision, electing to go to a site in Evanston, Illinois, which was given to it by Northwestern University. Reasons other than the free site were given for choosing Evanston, but none of these were unique.

(3) A subtle inhibiting factor was the growth of patient care within university medical centers and the growing town-gown problems. Because of increased specialization and the related complexity of resources necessary for the care of patients, consultation and complex treatment resources were gradually shifted to medical centers. It became increasingly apparent that the functioning of congenital heart diagnostic and surgical teams, endocrine and metabolic groups, infectious disease groups, and the like could not be carried on by solo practitioners any longer. New programs, such as the developing regional medical programs on heart disease, cancer, stroke, and related disorders, were designed in part to increase the effectiveness of the medical centers in relation to community resources in the interest of improved patient care.

With the trend toward maximum utilization of educational and community resources, private patients were cared for increasingly in university settings and many administrative complexities developed concerning the disposition of patient care fees. Patient care also contributed to the expansion which began with research and education staff increases. Many practitioners, viewing this expansion as a threat to their practices, opposed the trend. Associated with the complexities of patient care was the shift to a full-time faculty, which made inroads into the role of the individual practitioner on the medical school faculty. Many deans were preoccupied with town-gown problems and were very cautious about taking any public stand on health affairs which might be interpreted as opposition to the position of the AMA. The consideration of public policy related to health affairs therefore was circumspect to the point of inaction. (A study of the town-gown problem is reported lucidly by Dr. Patricia Kendall in "The Relationship Between Medical Educators and Medical Practitioners: Sources of Strain and Occasions for Cooperation in Educators and Practitioners as Factors in Medical and Health Care." [23] Dr. Anne Somers has also described this syndrome in "Conflict, Accommodation, and Progress: Some Socioeconomic Observations on Medical Education and the Practicing Profession." [24])

(4) The failure to incorporate faculty members into the mainstream of the Association was probably a major factor in reducing the influence of the AAMC within and without the medical centers. Medical educators were becoming increasingly professionalized, especially with the rapid growth of full-time clinical teachers. Although they had extra-institutional affiliations through national societies representing their disciplines, they had no representation in their roles as medical educators. The deans, on the numerous occasions when they discussed the transformation of the AAMC into an association of medical educators, rationalized that they represented the faculty members' interests. The faculty members certainly were not eager to press the point, for they had become skilled at lobbying for their interests through their informal extramural establishment in the study sections and advisory councils of the NIH. In addition, they had not been timid about developing some organizational structure for this establishment, for there had emerged Associations of Medical School Departmental Chairmen in medicine, surgery, pediatrics, psychiatry and so forth, which exerted considerable influence in Washington. After several years of discussion the Association voted to foster the development of an AAMC Council of Academic Societies, which would have representation on the Executive Council of the AAMC.[25] However this appeared to be locking the barn door after the horse was stolen, for each of these academic societies developed its own pattern of influencing policy related to its interests and needs; it was unlikely that they would forego their autonomy.

The preoccupation with research and growth in medical centers was resulting in improved care for the patient with complex or critical illness. The academic establishment, with its influence inside as well as outside the university, placed highest priority on the study and care of the hospitalized patient. (An example of the exercise of this priority may be observed in the establishment by the NIH in 1961 of a program of grants for clinical research centers. Initially these grants provided funds for the study of patients only while hospitalized. The funds could not be used to study the same patients as outpatients, a situation that created so many absurdities that the ruling was modified in 1965 to legitimize such outpatient studies.) This observation is presented, not with the objective of depreciating the significance of research on disease or patient care for the seriously ill patient, but rather to indicate that a lack of balance in planning for health education, research, and service was diverting public expenditures for health toward laboratory research with a concomitant lack of attention to the development of health services. This imbalance reflected a value system in which highest prestige was accorded laboratory investigations on hospitalized patients and little or no attention was given to the potentialities of the new research for keeping people well rather than treating them while sick. This could be thought of as a fixation on pathology rather than pathogenesis or a concern with disease as opposed to process and prevention. However we wish to view the problem, its practical effect was a neglect of outpatient services and the study of the delivery of health services. A few voices in medical education have recently been raised indicating that outpatient and community health services are a proper research interest for the medical schools.[26] It is interesting to observe that the academic establishment, made up of many people with broad social vision individually, has as a group been so silent on meeting the health needs of the people. My comment is made with the awareness that many meetings of medical educators have emphasized the importance of outpatient teaching. The fact remains that, except for small-scale innovations (comprehensive care clinics, home care programs, and so forth), there has been no reorganization of the delivery systems for care within university medical centers. In a later section, the reasons for this lack of reorganization are discussed more extensively. At this point I would only comment that sufficient attention will never be given to this problem until the preventive outpatient services are reinstitutionalized and given autonomy outside the existing departmental structure, for the existing departmental value system gives highest priority (and *properly* so) to the care of the sick.

The heavy emphasis on research supported by public expenditures along with the relative neglect of services was beginning to have an interesting and significant effect on the health record of the nation. Public health officials as well as legislators were becoming increasingly aware of the fact that the health record of the nation was not showing the much-hoped-for continuing improvement. This suggested that some efforts might be made in order to stimulate research and demonstration programs which might have a direct bearing on unresolved health problems (such as infant and maternal mortality, improved immunization rates, dental caries, effects of air pollution). Administratively these problems might be approached through contract research directed at a specific mission—an anathema to the academic establishment.[27] The academic establishment view was probably fortified by the awareness (accurate, no doubt) that such programs would compete with basic research for the research dollar. The establishment position defends the need for basic research unfettered by specific missions or controls (contract research). The academic establishment is then placed in an all or none position which is untenable. Those providing the support (the consumers) must at some point be destined to ask whether the research accomplishments were being applied in their interest.

The Second Quest for Normalcy

With the end of World War II the nation became engaged in a search for stability. The depression years were still fresh in the minds of many; the war years had been associated with some degree of enforced privation. The affluent society was growing, and one consequence seemed to be a general lack of interest in social legislation—culminating in the election of Eisenhower over Stevenson in 1952. As yet the nonaffluent population had not developed any articulate advocates or militancy of its own, and by the midfifties there was an active effort to intimidate social reformers through the McCarthy-led witch hunts.

The matter of improving medical care was not excepted in the lull in social legislation. Although President Truman was sensitive to the latent popular interest in a system of improving medical care by distributing its costs through an insurance plan, it was generally agreed that legislation for this purpose had little chance of being passed. The early drafts of congressional legislation in the late forties, although considered exploratory efforts by their sponsors—Wagner, Murray, and Dingell—were taken quite seriously by the AMA, which began to wage a major campaign against the Wagner-Murray-Dingell Bill. Regardless of protests to the contrary, the AMA became identified as a political-economic organization. The history of the transformation of the AMA into a political lobbying organization has been presented in considerable detail by Richard Harris.[28]

Because of its previous strong resistance to even voluntary insurance programs (or the corollary of support only for a fee-for-service transaction in rendering medical care with no intermediate third party) the AMA hierarchy viewed these legislative explorations with alarm. Previously it had relied largely on its intramural staff for the elaboration of political positions and action. The spokesman was the editor of the *Journal of the AMA,* Dr. Morris Fishbein. But by now the Association viewed the situation as sufficiently grave to reinforce its efforts. Taking a page in part from the California Medical Association, which had just waged a campaign against a state health insurance bill sponsored by Governor Warren, and in part from industry, they decided upon a campaign directed by a professional public relations firm. From this point on it became difficult to decipher how much policy was determined by public relations staff and how much by physician-members. In the process the leading professional spokesman for the organization, Dr. Fishbein, "retired" from the AMA in 1949.

As a result of the rigid opposition of the AMA to all open discussion, many physicians were sufficiently concerned to attempt a dialogue on the issues. A group of one hundred physicians publicly protested an assessment of $25 per year to finance the public relations program. The political power structure of the organization was in no mood for a dialogue; various threats to the careers of those who might dissent from the extreme and monolithic public position of the organization were common (the dependence of many physicians on membership in good standing in their medical societies for hospital appointments, board certifications, and other positions rendered them unusually vulnerable to coercion or threats thereof). The rise on the political ladder within the AMA was suited to eliminate dissent, for from county to state to national elections a screening process was in operation which made it virtually impossible for a dialogue on policy to develop at a higher level.

The hiring of a public relations staff had an effect on the staff of the organization as well as on the general membership. To outsiders it is difficult to comprehend that the AMA structure tends to form a closed society. Carter, in *The Doctor Business,* points out that one of the AMA's problems has been that the officers and staff *believe* their publicity releases.[29] It is probably more accurate to state that they act as though they believe the releases. Informal conversations with officers and staff indicate that there is much role playing and that in headquarters one plays by the rules of the game—which means playing it safe. In the process of writing speeches and copy for publications there is an assumption that the staff knows what the Board of Trustees thinks, and before long the Board of Trustees finds itself the author of statements on policy which have been generated by the staff within its headquarters. An example of this circularity in action is given in the following anecdote: In 1961 President Kennedy announced the appointment of a Presidential Panel on Mental Retardation. The charge to the Panel was such that opposition to it would have been akin to opposing motherhood. Much to the surprise of some of the AMA committees concerned with matters of mental retardation, the President of the AMA in a speech two weeks later announced AMA opposition to the Panel. On attempting to trace the origin of this position, the Director of Scientific Affairs of the AMA, found that the speech had been scheduled on another subject. The speech writer in public relations, on the assumption that if a Democratic president is *for* something the AMA automatically is *against* it, wrote into the speech an opposing policy position. Out of such stuff are policies born!

The closed system is not limited to staff. The various committees and councils in writing their reports seem to be preoccupied with what the Board of Trustees thinks. In this process there is a tendency to fantasy what the Board will find acceptable; as a result there is an inevitable looking backward to where the Board has been rather than to where it may be going. It becomes virtually impossible for the Board to receive recommendations for shifts in policy from its committees or staff.

In embracing a professional public relations approach assumed to be successful when employed by industry, the AMA was missing one ingredient: industry had a positive position in promoting a product; the AMA was only negative in opposing new legislation. Recognizing this lack, the public relations experts determined that the AMA should have a positive position on some issue and chose the support of voluntary hospital and health insurance, which the AMA had so vehemently opposed in the past. That this was a hollow, if not embarrassing, gesture was apparent from the fact that hospital and health insurance had already—in spite of the AMA's opposition—become widely accepted. Thus any new legislation was drafted on the assumption that such voluntary insurance was widely accepted and did not offer the fuller protection which was desired by many. Publicly the AMA was running to a position where many people had already been. In the meantime the advocates of a national health program recognized that various voluntary programs were refining their efforts and concentrating on legislation to meet more critical needs; in 1950 some of the first drafts of legislation for hospital and health insurance for elderly people were being formulated. The gradual refinement of this legislation and the buildup of its support was to go on for the next fifteen years in spite of the constant opposition of the AMA which offered few alternative legislative proposals until the final weeks prior to passage of the Medicare bill in 1965. Another example of the time lag in the AMA acceptance of social change was evident in its opposition in 1950 to the vendor medical payment (fee-for-service) provisions under public assistance; in the early 1960's the AMA embraced this approach as its own idea while attempting to stop Medicare through support of the Kerr-Mills legislation.

Insurance or Insolvency

But what had been happening to the consumer since World War II? The low-income consumer (generally referred to as "indigent") had few advocates, and services for him were undergoing a gradual deterioration by neglect. The more affluent groups were protecting themselves through a variety of voluntary insurance plans increasingly tied in with employment fringe benefits. Since availability of services was not a problem for the affluent group, it tended to focus its attention on the support of medical research (with the anticipation that the results would bring better health); the exploration of new patterns of delivering health services received little or no attention while support for research mounted. The emphasis on research, combined with the long years of repetition that the American people enjoyed the best health in the world, caused the public to neglect any thoroughgoing evaluation of the health status or services to the poor.

The growth of third-party payments (which include health insurance benefit payments, government expenditures, philanthropic expenditures, and the expenditures of employers to maintain industrial in-plant facilities) for personal health care expenditures (defined as hospital and nursing home care, services for professional personnel in private or group practice, school health services, industrial in-plant health services, and medical activities in federal units other than hospitals) reached 50.1 percent of the total health expenditure of $39,115,000,000 in 1966 in contrast to 35 percent of the total of $11 billion in 1950. Voluntary insurance was the source of 9 percent of all personal health care expenditures in 1950 and 25 percent in 1964. By 1964, 43 percent of the expenditures for the services of physicians in private practice were met by third-party payments. In spite of frequent representation against third-party payments by representatives of the AMA (these objections continued in connection with Part B [voluntary] payments for medical services after the passage of Medicare), data indicate that physicians with a gross annual income of $100,000 or more receive almost half their income from such sources while those grossing less than $20,000 receive one fourth of their income in this way.[30]

The orientation of all these plans was toward the payment for what has been termed "catastrophic illness" or hospital practice. Thus a subtle emphasis was placed on the hospitalization of patients, even when it might not be necessary, in order to spare the patient the cost of outpatient diagnostic services and professional fees. That the hospitalization plans (Blue Cross, Blue Shield, and private insurance firms) had become bureaucracies in their own right is evident from their many years of resistance to including outpatient diagnostic studies in their benefits. After years of exhorting physicians not to hospitalize patients for diagnostic studies which could be carried on in outpatient settings, the hospitalization plans gradually came to realize that this position was futile as long as hospitalization offered potent economic incentives to physician and patient.[31] Only when the plans realized that encouraging hospitalization put them in economic jeopardy did they modify their policies to include outpatient diagnostic studies.

The voluntary insurance plan payments for professional services also emphasized the catastrophic aspects of illness. The provisions for payments were based predominantly on surgical fee schedules. It was almost as though only surgeons had a hand in fee-schedule formulation, with a sop to nonsurgeons which authorized payment for hospital visits. Thus there were virtually no economic inducements to develop or to utilize preventive services among middle-income groups, who had to pay out of pocket for such services. It is possible that the development of surgically oriented fee schedules reflected the power structure as well as the traditional orientation of medicine. That this structure is changing is evident from the recent emergence of new organizations such as the Society of Internal Medicine and the Federation of Pediatric Societies, which have among their explicit aims the economic welfare of these practitioner groups and their patients, whose interests had been largely by-passed in insurance programs. Also families were increasingly asking for protection for office services (which they had been educated by the mass media to expect) rather than hospital care.

It is somewhat surprising that organized consumer groups— particularly organized labor, which was in the process of incorporating health insurance in its contracts as a fringe benefit— were so slow to recognize the defects inherent in this traditional approach to payment for health services. It was increasingly evident that provision for payment of surgical fees was a protection against major expenditures which did not necessarily result in the improvement of the quality of medical care. Indeed, several studies indicated that the incidence of some surgical procedures was inclined to go up presumably as a consequence of assured payment through insurance.[31, 32] Thus health insurance based on fee-for-service payment may have been having a paradoxical effect on the quality of care. Organized labor and other consumer groups began to think more actively about alternatives.

A major alternative was the development of prepayment programs to cover all health services, preventive as well as therapeutic. It was suggested that such programs would be too costly and that they could become insolvent. Historically such prepayment programs had survived financially; their difficulties lay in the strong opposition of the constituent medical societies of the AMA. In contrast the medical care section of the American Public Health Association had long been an advocate of prepaid group practice and provided some support for interested groups. The basic pattern of these programs was to employ physicians part time or full time to provide health services for their membership. The opposition of the medical societies took the form of denial of medical society membership, denial of hospital appointments, and other more subtle economic and professional punitive actions against the participating physician. This intransigence on the part of medical societies has continued to this day, and though there are some signs of softening of opposition in more overt ways, covert harassment of physicians working in prepayment plans still continues. This opposition has caused one of the leaders in American medicine, Dr. Robert Morison, until recently the Vice-President of the Rockefeller Foundation and now Director of the Division of Basic Biology at Cornell University, to comment, "the medical profession in the United States remains curiously preoccupied with private practice to a far greater extent than is true anywhere else in the world, except possibly Latin America. For some reason that is difficult for the outsider to grasp, the typical physician in the United States still feels that the only really honorable way to be paid is on a fee for service basis and that there is something just a little bit degrading about working for a salary—more than a little bit if the salary comes from the Government." [33] Perhaps the reason may not be so difficult to grasp when one considers the relatively higher fee structure for surgical procedures and the concomitantly high income. These are articulate, forceful people—witness the fact that their point of view is considered that of "the medical profession of the United States" by Dr. Morison even though 40 percent of the physicians in the United States are not in individual practice.

Although prepayment plans were attacked by organized medical societies as new and radical concepts, their roots go back to antiquity—antedating fee-for-service arrangements. In ancient China it was the custom for a physician to be paid only as long as he kept his patients well; if a patient became ill the physician was not to receive his fees. Prepayment plans provide an economic incentive to keep the patient well or to introduce preventive measures insofar as knowledge permits. (The specific problems of disease prevention will be dealt with in more detail later.) It is understandable therefore that some of the most imaginative comprehensive programs for early disease detection and for the evaluation of the quality and effectiveness— including cost effectiveness—of health services have been undertaken by prepayment groups.[34, 35] It is striking that few such programs have been undertaken by university medical centers or schools of public health, although the latter have provided contributions to the study of the financing of such programs.

As a consequence of medical society opposition, group practice prepayment health services have had a stormy course. The first such plan, organized by Dr. Michael Shadid, a practitioner in Elk City, Oklahoma, was subjected to years of harassment by the local and state medical societies. After some twenty years and a suit by the clinic against the medical society for restraint of trade, the society finally settled out of court and admitted the clinic physicians to membership. A more prominent conflict centered around the development of the Group Health Association prepayment plan for government employees in Washington, D. C. The Association had been organized in 1937, and for a period of time its physicians were subjected to pressures which almost drove it out of existence. Then, in 1943, an antitrust indictment of the AMA and the District of Columbia Medical Society was obtained by the Antitrust Division of the Department of Justice. The Supreme Court (in AMA vs. U.S.) found the AMA guilty of criminal action. In its opinion, the Court stated: "Professions exist because people believe they will be better served by licensing specially prepared experts to minister to their needs. The licensed monopolies which professions enjoy constitute in themselves severe restraints upon competition. But they are restraints which depend upon capacity and training, not privilege. Neither do they justify concerted criminal action to prevent the people from developing new methods of serving their needs. The people give the privilege of professional monopoly and the people may take it away." Since this judgment the national leadership has been more circumspect in its opposition and has cautioned local societies to exercise prudence. That such caution is not always heeded is evidenced by the continuing necessity for prepayment groups to bring court action against medical societies. In 1963 the Bellaire (Ohio) Medical Group instituted a lawsuit against the local medical society for excluding its physicians from membership. The suit was settled in 1965 with an agreement for binding, court-supervised arbitration in the event of future disputes over membership. In 1967 however the Group again had to resort to litigation in order to have the favorable award of the first arbitration proceeding enforced.

Prepayment plans continued to grow, albeit slowly, in spite of physicians working in such plans continuing to experience various types of harassment. One of the larger plans resulted from the health program developed for the workers in the ship-building division of the Kaiser Industries during World War II. This plan, which has its own hospitals, has functioned in a variety of communities in the Far West and is probably the most rapidly growing of the prepayment programs. The physicians in the plan work full time. In the East, the Health Insurance Plan of Greater New York has developed a membership of over 700,000, largely among city employees. This plan has explored various patterns of delivering services by utilization of full-time and part-time physicians throughout a large metropolitan complex; in the process it has acquired considerable data on the cost and effectiveness of services.

One of the most extensive comprehensive care prepayment programs was developed during the fifties under the auspices of the Health and Welfare Fund of the United Mine Workers. For example, the building of hospitals was part of the program, a necessary move because of the dearth of all health facilities in the mining areas. The United Mine Workers found the financing of hospitals precarious, as it had been for most groups in recent years. By 1964, because the plan was in financial difficulties due in part to the decline of the mining industry, the hospitals were turned over to other agencies. The increasing economic crisis resulting in considerable measure from automation in the mining industry also effected some reductions in the operation of the program. In more recent years, the Community Health Association of Detroit, with some impetus from the United Auto Workers, has been developing a prepayment program with an emphasis on preventive services and comprehensive care for families. On a smaller scale many other labor groups have been exploring new patterns of providing comprehensive health services, but many more have simply purchased available insurance programs.

The logic of developing comprehensive health services for families—regardless of the method of financing—is so overwhelming that the AMA is seemingly about to undergo some reversal in its position of persistent opposition. In its final report to the Board of Trustees of the AMA, the Citizens' Commission on Graduate Medical Education states:

It is time for decisive action to increase greatly the number of physicians who will devote their careers to the highly competent provision of comprehensive and continuing medical services. If organized medicine does not take the leadership in meeting this problem, others will. (p. 42)

The completely independent practice of medicine is no longer possible . . . Institutionalized practice in a hospital, a clinic, or some form of group practice, permits a higher quality of total service than the relatively independent practitioner can offer. A variety of skills, specialized knowledge in different areas, a more competent corps of paramedical aides, and expensive equipment that the solo practitioner can rarely afford are all brought together for the benefit of the patient who takes his medical problems to physicians based in a hospital or a group practice clinic. There are also advantages for the physician . . . (p. 25) [36]

Thus, some thirty-four years after the report of the Committee on the Costs of Medical Care, the advisors appointed by the AMA proffer similar counsel, and in the perspective of history perhaps thirty-four years is not a long time!

On Missing the Point

As general dissatisfaction with medical care became more apparent in the postwar period, various factors were suggested as the causes. Among them were two main points: (1) That there was a deterioration in the doctor-patient relationship, and that physicians should be better educated in psychiatry in order to gain a better understanding of the emotional problems of their patients. These criticisms were widely accepted (often uncritically) within and without the profession, at a time when the length of psychiatric education and its intensity were increasing. As dissatisfaction continued there were many who kept insisting that more and/or better psychiatric education was the answer. The persistence of the problem in spite of heroic teaching efforts did not clarify the issues fully. Some continued to blame the dehumanizing effect of scientific medicine, rather than the sociologic changes in medical practice such as increasing specialization and subspecialization and increasing mobility of our population, resulting in discontinuity in care (it is estimated that 20 percent of our population moves each year). Although better psychiatric teaching is always in order, it is an oversimplification to suggest it as a panacea. Note that those who long for the doctor-patient relationship of yesteryear generally refer to the "old" family doctor (never the "young" family doctor). What they long for is the wisdom gained from a lifetime of practice and continuity in patient care; although psychiatric knowledge and teaching have advanced, they cannot replace clinical experience for the young physician. An anecdote told by Dr. William Sodeman illustrates this difference: In the twenties a patient with lobar pneumonia entering a hospital had a 30 percent chance of dying; if he survived, he was critically ill for ten days until a "crisis" occurred, and he remained in the hospital for a month or longer—often with debilitating complications. If he recovered, generally a good doctor-patient relationship resulted. Today a patient rarely dies, is treated with antibacterial drugs, and often leaves the hospital in two days, stating to the resident physician on his way out, "But, Doctor, I didn't quite get your name." [37]

(2) That the decline in general practitioners was due to the seduction by medical school faculty of medical students from careers in general practice to the specialties. This resulted in faculty exhortation (perhaps defensive) of students to enter general practice and in numerous efforts to improve the image of the general physician. The American Academy of General Practice was organized to improve the lot of general physicians and to proselytize more actively. In spite of all efforts, it is apparent that exhortation is not the answer. Indeed, among general physicians many seem to be giving up their general practices to return to training for the specialties. It would appear that the functions assumed by general physicians in the past will gradually need to be assumed by new patterns of care—unless this steady downward trend can be reversed, and this does not seem likely. Thus we come face to face with meeting the needs of the consumer in a fashion designed for the latter third of the twentieth century.

It is appropriate therefore that we turn our attention to the consumer of health services. Without an advocate in the medical practitioner establishment (the AMA), the medical school establishment (the AAMC) or the medical research establishment (the new culture of medical research workers), what has been his fate?

3 The Consumer Revolution: Translating

Knowledge into Programs (1960–1968)

Status 1960

By 1960 the impact of population mobility and social change on the health of the people could not be denied. Rapid urbanization was associated with an accentuation of rural poverty and lack of rural services, while intensifying the decay of the cities; the poor—urban and rural—became poorer. The struggle for human rights through the civil rights movement highlighted the nation's long-term neglect of these social and economic problems. Small wonder that the President-elect in 1960 sounded a challenge: "Ask not what your country can do for you; ask what you can do for your country."

The long neglect was perhaps nowhere more apparent than in the field of health. No longer could the platitudes that we had the best health record in the world or that our system of health services was the best obtainable be offered without serious challenge. Those charged with guarding the public's health realized that infant mortality rates were no longer declining significantly; in 1958 the rate rose slightly for the first time. The relative position of the United States in infant mortality had dropped to sixteenth among the nations of the world (figure 4). It was clear that this problem reflected the higher mortality rates among the poor, especially the nonwhite poor (figure 5); the relative disadvantage of the poor by any health criterion was becoming apparent to public health officials (figure 6).[1]

Another source of concern was the gradual deterioration of the public hospital system, which had undergone little updating in its physical structures or its staffing patterns since its

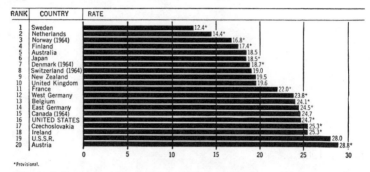

RANK	COUNTRY	RATE
1	Sweden	12.4*
2	Netherlands	14.4*
3	Norway (1964)	16.8*
4	Finland	17.4*
5	Australia	18.5
6	Japan	18.5*
7	Denmark (1964)	18.7*
8	Switzerland (1964)	19.0
9	New Zealand	19.5
10	United Kingdom	19.6
11	France	22.0*
12	West Germany	23.8*
13	Belgium	24.1*
14	East Germany	24.5*
15	Canada (1964)	24.7
16	UNITED STATES	24.7*
17	Czechoslovakia	25.3*
18	Ireland	25.3*
19	U.S.S.R.	28.0
20	Austria	28.8*

*Provisional.

Fig. 4. Infant mortality rates (number of deaths under 1 year of age per 1000 live births), selected countries, 1965.
SOURCE: J. B. Richmond, "The Gap in Child Health Care," *The American Federationist 74*:11 (November 1967).

inception in the eighteenth century. Public outpatient services also had undergone little change over the decades, consequently disillusioning the poor, who are dependent on its services. For large numbers of the poor—if they were fortunate enough to live close to a hospital—the hospital's emergency room was the main source of medical care. In a study of Ohio hospitals which seems characteristic of the trend throughout the country, it was found that emergency room visits had increased from 6 to 10 percent per year since World War II (figure 7).[2] There is no evidence that this trend will lessen. For many in rural areas almost no services were readily available.

The distribution of health services on the basis of the open marketplace accentuated the lack of services to the poor. Physicians fled the slums, as well as the areas of rural poverty, for the more affluent suburbs. Indeed they had no choice if they were to survive economically. Thus in South Boston, where there were 39 physicians in 1942, there were only 19 in 1964—in spite of a rising population. In Chicago the poverty areas were found to have half the number of medical practitioners per 1,000 persons that the nonpoverty areas have.[3] Thus an economist, Herman Somers, in commenting on the objectives of health insurance programs, stated, "If there are resulting shortages, few would advocate that a selection of who is to be served be based on

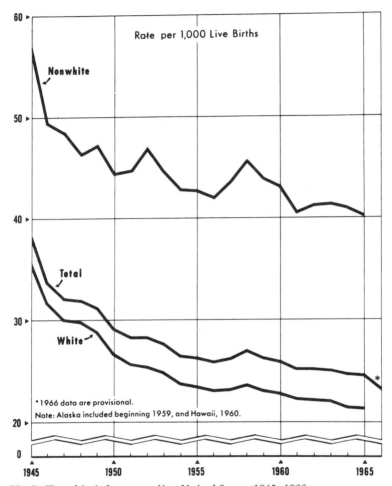

Fig. 5. Trend in infant mortality, United States, 1945–1966.
SOURCE: *Statistical Bulletin*, vol. 48. Metropolitan Life Insurance Co.,
May 1967.

capacity to make direct out-of-pocket payments." Although few
might publicly advocate such a policy, the nation endorsed it,
because the affluent could purchase the range of services at their
need and pleasure while the health of the poor was unattended

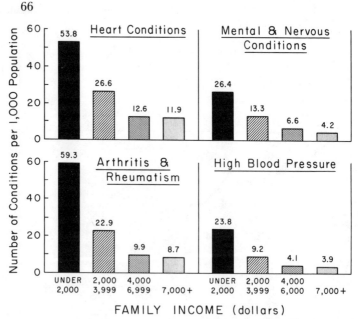

Fig. 6. Disease categories and family income.
SOURCE: "Medical Care Status and Family Income," *Chronic Illness and Disability*. Washington, D. C.: National Center for Health Statistics, May 1964, p. 60.

in any systematic way. The same economist goes on to say, "Surely, equity demands that, whatever the state of adequacy of medical facilities and manpower, the aged, the disabled, and the poor have access reasonably equal to those of other citizens." [4] Many may argue defensively that welfare vendor payments for medical care entitled welfare patients to equal care. But the inadequate fee schedules have increased the shortage of physicians available for such services, and the generally dehumanizing aspects of the establishment of welfare eligibility and its constant scrutiny have not encouraged welfare clients to use these services—to say nothing of preventive services. The so-called "gray zone" patient, between welfare and economic adequacy, generally found himself with nowhere to turn. The re-

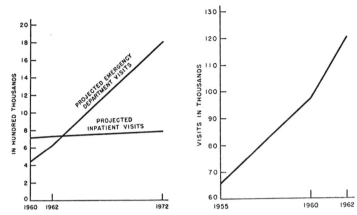

Fig. 7. Growth of emergency department visits: (left) projected emergency department and inpatient visits in selected Ohio urban hospitals, 1960 to 1972; (right) growth of emergency department visits in rural hospitals in Ohio, 1955 to 1962.
SOURCE: V. D. Seifert and J. S. Johnstone, "Meeting the Emergency Department Crisis," *Hospitals, JAHA* (Nov. 1, 1966).

cent passage of Title 19 of the Social Security Amendments may help this group, although some of the states are becoming so restrictive in their income eligibility standards that eligibility may not far exceed existing welfare standards.

The old cliché that only the very rich and the very poor receive excellent medical care might have been true, but only for very critical illnesses for the poor—and then only if they lived near a hospital and could gain admission. In some areas the possibility of their gaining admission might be based on criteria other than illness—race, for example. Thus a double standard of medical care had grown up in the United States in the face of our complacency about what was gratuitously called "the best system of medical care in the world." Although there were studies and recommendations for a national health program (particularly notable were the timely recommendations of the President's Commission on the Health Needs of the Nation named by President Truman in 1951 [5]) the Hill-Burton Legislation for hospital construction, the provision for vendor medical payments under public assistance in the 1950 amendments to the Social Security Act, and the increasing NIH appropriations for research were the only major health legislation since the thirties.

It was apparent that the professional health establishments had no plan for changing this situation which was approaching crisis proportions. The AMA was devoting all of its resources and energy to the defeat of the pending Medicare legislation; the public health officers and schools of public health of the nation—in spite of the embarrassingly unfortunate public health statistics and the increasing pollution of our water and air—had no major proposals; the medical education and research establishment was busy with its pursuit of new medical knowledge unconcerned about meeting the health needs of the people; and the federal health agencies, particularly the Public Health Service, had virtually no program of medical services for the poor or for the nation at large. The growth of hospital and health insurance, fragmented as it was, was giving the consumer some sense of his potential for meeting his medical care needs. Nevertheless insurance was held by only the more articulate and influential consumer, and the poor remained without an advocate.

A Personalized Approach: The Kennedy Years

It was into this situation that President Kennedy entered in 1961. He acknowledged the significance of the long years of neglect by developing a Message to Congress on health and later on mental health. Since the forces for Medicare legislation for elderly people were continuing their efforts, his support served as a catalyst. It became apparent that widespread support and the obvious need and logic of the program made it only a matter of time before the legislation was passed over the opposition of the AMA. In the process the representatives of the consumers, the members of Congress, were becoming more sophisticated concerning the relative lack of health services for people and approaches to improving these services.

It was apparent from the State of the Union Message that the President had no overall design for a health program. He expressed concern for such obvious neglect as our failure to immunize many of our young children. And, perhaps because of his personal interest in the problems of mental retardation, probably a consequence of a sister's affliction, he proposed that these problems receive adequate attention. Toward this end he appointed a presidential panel of experts and citizens-at-large to study and to make recommendations concerning the retarded. This panel made its report in 1963 [6] and steps were taken to translate its recommendations into action through the enactment of the Mental Retardation Facilities Construction Act in 1963. This legislation represented a fragmented approach even to the problems of mental retardation, for the causes of mental retardation are many, and preventive and therapeutic efforts depend upon a more general health program. Nevertheless in the face of great need for all health services, the planning for clinical facilities for the mentally retarded represented a practical step forward.

The new President was also concerned about the care of the psychiatric patient. This is a problem of great magnitude in human—as well as financial—terms; approximately one out of every two hospitalized patients in the United States occupies a psychiatric-hospital bed. The quality of service in these hospitals had declined to such a point that the President referred to the "warehousing" of the mentally ill.[7] Most of these hospitals were state supported, so they reflected the financial problems of the states after World War II. The President's concern was translated into a public program through the Community Mental Health Centers Act of 1963. Again this represented a fragmented approach to the problems of mental health, separating them from a comprehensive health program. These programs for Community Mental Health Centers and Mental Retardation Facilities Construction remained ill-defined as they developed—a good example of how our humanitarian concerns may outstrip our knowledge for action. To this day there is no clear concept of how the Community Mental Health Center will improve the mental health of our people! Since most mental health services have served primarily the middle class, there has been little experience with extending such services to low-income groups. There is some conviction that an extensive network of community-based services may minimize admissions to psychiatric hospitals, but no one yet knows what the balance between hospitalized and nonhospitalized patients optimally should be to serve the interests of society and the individual person.

Yet another fragmented approach was under way to deal with problems of heart disease, cancer, and stroke. Anecdote has it that this legislation "began when Mrs. Kennedy started to redecorate the interior of the White House and asked for donations of furniture and pictures. One of the donors, so the story goes, gave so many excellent things that President and Mrs. Kennedy asked if they could do something for the donor in return. The answer was, please do something to conquer cancer.

"Plans began to go forward, so it is said, to establish a presidential commission on cancer and heart disease. The latter was added perhaps out of concerns elsewhere in the executive branch. Stroke was added when President Kennedy's father became ill. Thus, the 'killer-diseases' concept came into being and was passed on to the new president." [8]

With the untimely death of President Kennedy, President Johnson pursued this approach to a health program and announced early in 1964, in a message to Congress, that he was appointing a Commission on Heart Disease, Cancer, and Stroke. The Commission was appointed on March 7, 1964, under the chairmanship of a distinguished surgeon, Dr. Michael E. DeBakey; by December, 1964, its final report was submitted to the President. This was a very comprehensive consideration of the problems facing the nation in connection with these disorders; the Commission was not timid in translating its concerns into thirty-five recommendations. Only three of the recommendations formed the basis for legislative consideration in the House and Senate:

Recommendation 1. The Commission recommends the establishment of a national network of Regional Heart Disease, Cancer and Stroke Centers for clinical investigation, teaching *and patient care,* in universities, hospitals and research institutes and other institutions across the country.

Recommendation 2. The Commission recommends the establishment of a national network of *Diagnostic and Treatment Stations* in communities across the nation, to bring the highest medical skills in heart disease, cancer and stroke within reach of every citizen.

Recommendation 3. The Commission recommends that a broad and flexible program of grant support be undertaken to stimulate the formation of medical complexes whereby university medical schools, hospitals, and other health care and research agencies and institutions work in concert.[9] (Italics mine)

It was clear that the Commission was concerned about patient care as well as research and education. That the forces shaping health legislation were not ready to explore such new patterns of meeting the consumer's needs is apparent from the subsequent legislative history of the bills introduced for consideration by the House and Senate. The various establishments with potent lobbies, such as the AMA and the American Hospital Association, were joined by the voluntary health organizations such as the American Cancer Society and the American Heart Association to defer any action that would alter existing patterns of patient care. For example, in his testimony, the President of the American Heart Association, Dr. Carleton B. Chapman, stated: "The American Heart Association is very much in agreement with the main objective of the proposal, which is basically to make it possible for the Nation's physicians to provide our people with the best possible diagnosis and treatment of heart disease and stroke. But for the proposal to accomplish this high aim, the development must proceed according to an orderly sequence; and the first step is, beyond question, *to expand and improve the clinical training programs* of our country's medical schools and affiliated hospitals. Full development of categorical centers and community stations must inevitably be delayed until the people to man them are available." [8] (Italics mine)

The focus on education and training as a prerequisite to any expansion or reorganization of services serves (especially on the part of politically vulnerable public officials) as a delaying tactic. Although logic seems so much on the side of this approach, in fact progress rarely occurs in so orderly a fashion in a democratic society. Evidence would indicate that the establishment of a working program with related financial support and jobs, serves as the most forceful stimulus for the expansion of training programs. The vast expansion of educational and training programs in the health field in the early days of World War II is a dramatic example of our potentialities when we are convinced of need and have support.

By the time the bills emerged for final presentation and passage they had undergone considerable transformation. The Commission had a concept of thirty-five regional complexes to provide more adequate care (along with research and education) for those afflicted with heart disease, cancer, stroke and related disorders. But when the bill was passed in 1965 by the eighty-ninth Congress (P.L. 89–239), the objectives had become:

Through grants to encourage and assist in the establishment of regional cooperative arrangements among medical schools, research institutions, and hospitals for *research and training* (including continuing education) and for related demonstrations of patient care in the fields of heart disease, cancer, stroke, and related diseases;

To afford to the medical profession and the medical institutions of the nation, through such cooperative arrangements, the opportunity of making available to their patients the latest advances in the diagnosis and treatment of these diseases; and

By these means to improve generally the health, manpower and facilities available to the nation, and to accomplish these ends *without interfering with the patterns, or with the methods of financing, of patient care or professional practice,* or with the administration of hospitals and in cooperation with practicing physicians, medical center officials, hospital administrators, and representatives from appropriate voluntary health agencies. (Italics mine)

Thus the provisions for patient care were specifically excluded; and the entry of a patient into the system of the regional program was to be through a practitioner of medicine. The plan for a finite number of model centers was now revised to permit any number of medical centers to become applicants for program funds. The innovative aspects of the program are currently being developed with the help of planning grants. Some of the unique features of the program are (1) the development of programs on a geographically functional basis rather than on the basis of political boundaries or jurisdictions; (2) the stimulus for health agencies and institutions in a region to collaborate if grants are to be awarded; (3) the stimulus to plan, develop, and utilize expensive and elaborate resources in a region on a practical basis (if left to professionals on a competitive basis there is a tendency to duplicate unnecessarily such costly programs as open heart surgical teams and artificial kidney programs for which personnel are scarce); (4) cooperative training programs for all health personnel with particular emphasis on training new health aides to assist the health professionals; and (5) the exploration of new programs of continuing education for health professionals—especially physicians. This last provision may well prove to be the most important area of the program, providing for the first time adequate resources for utilizing new techniques in teaching and communication. Particularly effective in the educational process are those techniques which can be used in the physician's daily care of patients. Space does not permit a detailed discussion of the problems of continuing education for physicians. (Its many difficulties have been well summarized in a publication by Dr. George Miller.[10]

A fascinating description of the inroads which pharmaceutical manufacturers have made in this`field is presented by Dr. Charles May.[11])

Although the financing of patient care is specifically exempt, the passage of Medicare legislation (Title 18) and legislation to finance medical care for those unable to pay (Title 19) makes it feasible for more people to receive care. Perhaps the most significant aspect of the program is the drawing together of citizens and professionals, representing institutions as well as the general public, to plan for a given region, because any national health program will inevitably depend upon regionalization of services. Although the legislative limitations on the program for heart disease, cancer, stroke, and related diseases continue the fragmentation of health services, the scope of the program is broad enough to include many of man's ills (patients with diagnoses of heart disease, cancer, and stroke accounted for 25 percent of the time spent by patients in short-term general hospitals in 1962 [9]). But as in the development of health insurance, the greatest emphasis was placed on sickness rather than on health, in spite of the possibilities for development of preventive services under the authorization of the Act. Thus, what started out as a bold, exploratory venture to bring services to the consumer, ended as a program which will bring him benefits by indirection.

Programmatic Approaches

As the midsixties approached, it was apparent that the increasing sophistication of Congress in matters of health and increasing pressures for social legislation would change the emphasis of health proposals from concern for specific organs and diseases to consideration of a broader health program. The personal interest of the late President Kennedy had heightened the nation's awareness of its needs in health and prepared the way for the broader background necessary for new programs.

A major concern of the nation, articulated during the Kennedy administration and continued into the Johnson administration, was the problem of poverty—and its intensification—in the most affluent period of our history. Due to the pragmatism of a democratic society, no overall blueprint emerged; instead a series of Acts, which pointed to new directions, were passed by Congress. To deal with the problems of poverty across a broad front, the Economic Opportunity Act (P.L. 88–452) was passed, setting up a new agency (Office of Economic Opportunity) under the Executive Office of the President. In addition to his general antipoverty functions, the director of the agency was instructed to conduct programs in various fields "including employment, job training and counseling, health, vocational rehabilitation, etc . . ." and in so doing to consider such factors as "school dropout rates, military service rejection rates . . . the incidence of disease, disability and infant mortality; housing conditions; adequacy of community facilities and services; and the incidence of crime and juvenile delinquency." Social Security Act amendments were adopted to extend maternal- and child-health services for the poor; and in education, Congress enacted the Elementary and Secondary Education Act in 1965 (P.L. 89–10), Title I of which was aimed at improving the education of the poor.

The new health programs of the Children's Bureau explored new ways to develop services for maternal, infant, and child care for the poor. The Office of Economic Opportunity through its community action program undertook a comprehensive summer program combining educational, welfare, and health services for children about to enter school in the fall of 1965 (Project Head Start). That this program tapped a latent community interest in the development of disadvantaged children was evidenced by the response. Within a few months 2,690 communities provided facilities and programs for half (560,000) of the nation's poor children about to enter school. From the review of the health records of the children, existing knowledge about the lack of health services for young children was further documented; practically none had experienced continuing health supervision, and evidence of earlier dental care was unusual. Strangely enough, many of the medical societies which for years had claimed that our health services were adequate, were now complaining that they were being asked to take on an impossible load. In spite of many problems, health workers were remarkably effective in providing care for children who had been long neglected. But obviously this was another fragmented program which was necessary because the poor had no systematic, continuing health services. Certainly the children in Project Head Start (and those poor children who were not enrolled) should have been the recipients of care from the prenatal period on.

A Bumper Crop of Health Legislation

The Eighty-ninth Congress, in 1965, passed more health legislation than had been passed in any previous session; in addition to the Heart Disease, Cancer and Stroke Amendments of 1965 for regional medical programs, it passed the Title 18 and Title 19 amendments of the Social Security Act (Medical Assistance, P.L. 89–97). These were probably the most far-reaching measures concerning the financing of medical care yet enacted in the United States.

The fifty years of debate over health insurance, the rising costs of hospital and medical care, and to some extent the intensity of the AMA's efforts to oppose any form of federal legislation* all served to increase consumer (and congressional) awareness, interest, and support, so there was little doubt that the legislation would pass. The forces set in motion in open support of the proposed bills during the Kennedy years gained momentum during the Johnson administration, and it was only

* This opposition continued until the very last days of the legislative battle, when the AMA advocated "Eldercare" in opposition to Medicare as a last resort—a stand which did not rally much support, since even "friendly" congressmen felt that if the AMA could support such legislation now, it was ludicrous not to have done so in the past.

a matter of time. Although the AMA considered the passage of the bills a congressional betrayal, there seemed to be no doubt that Congress was reacting to consumer (voter) support.

The Medicare legislation (Title 18) provided every person 65 or older—except retired federal employees, who are covered by the Federal Employees Health Benefits Act—with 60 days of hospital care, after a standard $40 deductible provision presumably to avoid unnecessary hospitalization; 30 more days of hospital care at a charge of $10 a day; 20 days of free nursing-home care; 80 more days of nursing-home care at a charge of $5 a day; 100 home visits by nurses or other health specialists after hospitalization; and 80 percent of the cost of hospital diagnostic tests, after a $20 deductible provision for each series. To pay for this, the taxable wage base of the Social Security system was raised to $6,600 a year, and the tax itself was increased by one half of 1 percent for both employee and employer. A voluntary supplement provided for payment of 80 percent of what the bill called "reasonable charges" for all physicians' services, after a $50-a-year deductible provision; another 100 home visits, whether a patient had been hospitalized or not; and the costs of nonhospital diagnostic tests, surgical dressings, splints, and rented medical equipment. To pay for this coverage, people 65 or older who wished to participate were each to contribute $3 a month, and their contributions were to be supplemented by a matching sum from the Treasury's general revenues—both amounts being subject, as were the other cost-sharing provisions, to revision in future years if costs rose appreciably.*

An analysis of the provisions of Titles 18 and 19 causes some wonder at the intensity of organized medicine's opposition to the legislation. The provisions are basically for the financing of hospital and medical care; there is no provision for any change in the delivery systems for medical care. (In 1967 the Social Security Amendments added research funds to Medicare for ex-

* In 1968 the contribution was increased to $4 per month by congressional action.

perimentation with delivery and financing and added a free-choice provision to Medicaid to cover payments outside of the fee-for-service pattern.) Interpretatively, one may observe that an interesting social dynamic had occurred: the architects of the Social Security Amendments, while innovative concerning financing, had accepted for the time being the existing pattern of delivering medical care. Thus the long years of emphasis on fee-for-service arrangements by the AMA, as contrasted to pre-payment programs, had its effect even upon its adversaries. This is not meant to imply that the Medicare advocates were oblivious to other patterns; they had to judge what was politically feasible.

Because a high proportion of the health expenditure is for hospital services (see figure 3), the Medicare legislation properly places emphasis on the financing of such services. But it provides relatively few potent stimuli or incentives for the reorganization, extension, and quality improvement in the services. Unless local consumer pressures develop, the incentives are weak indeed for the development of more and better home care services and more adequate nursing-home and convalescent care facilities. Within the hospitals themselves more imaginative approaches to bed-utilization review will become necessary if such a review is to be other than a perfunctory approval of existing practices. Although coverage for outpatient services provides some incentive for the conservation of hospital beds, the fact that this coverage is only partial (80 percent) for visits to the physician's office and is associated with a twenty-dollar deductible provision for each series of tests tends to minimize the use of these services by groups needing them most.

The partial coverage for various services under Medicare and the deductible clauses undoubtedly stemmed from a desire for fiscal soundness, but these provisions place the burden on those least able to afford services. For the more affluent groups the provisions are not a significant hardship. Thus the poor remain proportionately at a disadvantage. It is also appropriate to note that the deductible features are a deterrent to the development of preventive and early diagnostic programs, particularly for the low income groups who need such services the most. The reasoning behind deductible clauses seems to be that, if health services are available, they will be overutilized and abused—an idea which has never been substantiated. (Those who have tried to develop community-wide programs in diabetes, tuberculosis, or cancer control know very well that the problem is really the opposite: it takes much health education to get people to utilize services properly and adequately.) The abuse approach, followed to its logical conclusion, would assume that wealthy persons would be deluging physicians' offices because cost is no factor. Although there may be hypochondriacs, rich as well as poor, demand for service is an individual matter; the poor as a group should not have to suffer reduced accessibility of service because of the hypochondria or misuse of services by a few.

The lack of provision for periodic health examinations, screening programs for early disease detection, and eye examinations also indicates some of the limitations of the program. The lack of incentives for reorganizing health services through the exploration of comprehensive-care programs based on group practice indicates the extent to which Medicare has accepted traditional patterns. Medicare does nothing to encourage a redistribution of professional services to areas which have great shortages. Small wonder that a nonmedical observer of the medical scene, John Dunlop of Harvard, was moved to comment, "The real function of the cost increases of the past decade, and those in process, should be to compel vast structural changes in the organization of medical care. Nothing could be worse in our society today than to say we need another three or five billion dollars for medical care, and then simply duplicate or multiply the arrangements that we now have. That would get us nowhere." [12]

The pumping of more money into existing systems of care is also apparent in the companion legislation to Medicare—Title 19 of the Social Security Amendments. As a deterrent to the development of Medicare, the AMA had supported legislation for medical assistance to the aged (Kerr-Mills bill) which passed in 1960. This legislation provided for assistance to states which elected to match federal funds; thus the poor states tended not to participate, although the number of participants had increased to thirty-six states, the District of Columbia, Guam, Puerto Rico, and the Virgin Islands by 1964. The requirement of a means test also minimized utilization, even in states which were participating. Title 19 represented an extension of the Kerr-Mills program to the needy of some additional age groups; (it excludes single people and couples who are not parents of dependent children, blind, disabled or aged;) again however the program was contingent on matching federal with state funds, with the more affluent states receiving a smaller percentage of matching funds. Each state was required to provide benefits by 1975, and each state was to define eligibility, thus paving the way for a wide variety of programs. The differences in the criteria for eligibility among the states is already becoming apparent: New York's legislature, for example, originally specified an annual income of $6,000 or less for a family of four as the level of eligibility as compared to a level of approximately $3,500 in Michigan. The 1967 legislation on Title 19 limits income eligibility to 133⅓ percent of welfare assistance payments. In many states this would bring Title 19 income eligibility below the poverty line—a major step backward.

However Title 19 provides only for the financing of care; it does nothing about providing incentives for the recruitment of professional health personnel for poverty areas. Thus one result of the program could be a deterioration in the quality of care, caused by physicians in poverty areas seeing many more patients than they did before.[13] Title 19 provides no incentives for the development of preventive services. For example, many states will not use these funds to reimburse free standing-clinics and public health facilities which often make preventive services available for the poor. In many states this program will not be a significant improvement over the prevailing welfare vendor payments on a fee-for-service basis.

In 1965 the Health Professions Educational Assistance Amendments (P.L. 89–290) were also passed providing funds for direct assistance to medical centers for the education of students in the health professions. Although the original legislation was passed in 1963 (the Health Professions Assistance Act [P.L. 88–129]) no funds were appropriated except for the Health Professions Student Loan Program; thus the amendments constituted a significant development in providing direct assistance to medical education for operational as well as construction purposes. This legislation was very similar to that which had been introduced in 1948 and which passed the Senate; however, it never reached the point of hearings in the House of Representatives. The Executive Council of the AAMC had supported the legislation in 1948, but it apparently had not done sufficient background work in gathering support from university officers, for the opposition of the AMA lobby combined with the lack of support of some university presidents served to prevent the consideration of the bill by the House of Representatives. By 1963 the officers of the universities and medical centers were in agreement that such legislation was desirable.

Notes on Fragmentation

By 1965 increasing consumer interest had begun to highlight the lack of coordinated effort and national planning in health service programs. This lack of coordination was particularly disturbing in the face of constantly rising expenditures and absence of continuing improvement in some aspects of the national health record (see figures 4,5,6). The shortages of health personnel, while most dramatic in poverty areas, were also evident to some degree in more affluent areas, where complaints were frequent concerning the overwork of physicians and the difficulty of making appointments. Nursing services were in short supply almost everywhere. But the shortages were always disproportionately greater for the poor.

In the light of these problems and the dearth of comprehensive proposals for dealing with them, Congress—its sophistication considerably increased with respect to health issues through the long debates on Medicare—undertook a review of our national health problems. In April, 1965, the House Committee on Interstate and Foreign Commerce directed its Special Subcommittee on HEW Investigation to study "the huge, expanding and farflung operations of the Department and of the governmental machinery and procedures used to coordinate the health programs, both within the Department and with agencies outside the Department having substantial health responsibilities." [14,15] In his introductory remarks at the hearings, the Chairman of the Subcommittee, Congressman Paul G. Rogers, stated, "Lack of communication, overlapping of responsibility, interagency rivalry, and lack of coordination among Federal, State, and local health authorities will only dilute our energies and hamper our efforts to achieve better health for all our citizens." [14]

To care for specific health needs, a variety of categorical programs had grown up over the years—each with good reason. But as in any large organization, there was a tendency for "hardening of the categories" to set in. Thus some programs were based on disease (tuberculosis, venereal diseases, cancer, mental illness, and so forth), some on age (Medicare, maternal and child health services and others), some on institutions (for example, school health services and welfare medical services), some on geographic or political jurisdictions (such as state and local health departments and Appalachian Regional Council programs), some on income (poverty health programs, welfare medical programs)—or on combinations of categories (such as the Regional Medical Programs for Heart Disease, Cancer, Stroke and Related Diseases and Crippled Childrens' Services). Small wonder that one of the major recommendations in the Report of the Special Subcommittee was that "There is a need to develop comprehensive health planning for the Nation's health effort; establishment of a National Health Council." [15]

By 1966 the concern over fragmentation had reached a point

at which a new legislative approach was thought to be necessary. This took the form of a Comprehensive Health Planning Act (P.L. 89–749) which charged the states with planning for health programs on a programmatic rather than a categorical basis. This act placed the responsibility for planning on existing departments and/or new state agencies set up for this purpose. It thus emphasizes the political boundaries of the states, although there is authorization for area wide planning among the states. The integration of interstate programs with state programs is to be accomplished in the interest of the public health. The coordination of the regional medical programs for heart disease, cancer, stroke, and related diseases which are not tied to political boundaries remains to be accomplished. In many states health departments have been charged with this responsibility, and these departments have difficulty in recruiting and retaining competent personnel and have been subjected traditionally to various pressures; it therefore remains to be seen whether they can lead the way to innovative planning. Nevertheless a new dimension in planning for health has been introduced by the legislative requirement that at least 51 percent of the members of the Board of any such agency be consumers.

Not all of the problems of fragmentation could be attributed to sources of financing or to administrative auspices. The progress in medicine, particularly the development of specialization —and subspecialization—was making comprehensive medical care increasingly difficult to obtain.

Consumer Voices

Since few medical voices were heard in favor of developing new ways to meet the health needs of the people, it was logical that nonmedical groups would interest themselves in a problem which was building up to crisis proportions.

In an effort to respond to the needs of the poor for continuing, comprehensive health services provided under group auspices, the Office of Economic Opportunity in 1965 attempted to stimulate communities—in collaboration with existing medical institutions such as medical schools; health departments; hospitals; medical, dental, and other professional societies; and local antipoverty agencies—to develop neighborhood health centers for low-income groups.[16] This program is a family care plan which has as its function the development of an institutional system to provide services formerly performed by the general physician. In addition to providing health services for the poor, the program offers an institutional vehicle for redistributing scarce health manpower, such as physicians, by making it possible for them to work in low-income neighborhoods and survive economically.[17]

The matter of redistributing personnel and redefining their functions—particularly by providing assistants of various kinds—is a major issue in any consideration of health manpower. One may raise the question, for example, whether attracting physicians to work in the poor neighborhoods of the large cities may drain the suburban areas of services. However the corollary question is whether the suburban areas can undergo some reduction in health personnel without any deterioration in their health records because of their favorable ecology, which reflects their better socio-economic status. Certainly poor housing, crowding, poor diet, and inadequate hygienic circumstances—in addition to inadequate medical care—contribute to the poor health record of the low-income group.

The neighborhood health center program made it possible to explore the utilization of nonprofessional personnel in some of the functions traditionally performed by professionals. These centers provided opportunities for the adequate utilization of nonprofessionals in preventive programs, including health education. This program was designed for the poor, but its implications for health services for the general population are apparent.

Although a comprehensive care program seems an added financial burden, studies indicate that the per capita health expenditures (nonhospital) for 1965 were approximately $140 per year. The program of comprehensive care in neighborhood health centers can be accomplished for approximately the same amount. Of course this would necessitate administrative rearrangements for funding, so that monies now being expended in a variety of ways could be channeled into such a program of comprehensive care. This program also stipulates that consumers (neighborhood residents) be involved in establishing the policies for such centers, in an effort to maintain responsiveness to community needs and to minimize the possibility that the new clinics will replicate the inadequacies of existing clinics for the poor. The old clinics have been described by Dr. Alonzo Yerby as follows:

The pervasive stigma of charity permeates our arrangements for health care for the disadvantaged, and whether the program is based upon the private practice of medicine or upon public or non-profit clinics and hospitals, it tends to be piecemeal, poorly supervised, and uncoordinated. Those who provide the services tend to focus their attention on the episode of disease or even the symptom, defending their actions on the grounds that they are poorly paid by the public welfare agency, or that their mission of teaching and research must come first.

In most of our large cities, the hospital out-patient department together with the emergency room, is the basic source of care for the poor. Today's out-patient departments still retain some of the attributes of their predecessors, the 18th Century free dispensaries. They are crowded, uncomfortable, lacking in concern for human dignity and to make it worse, *no longer free.*

To these unhappy circumstances has been added a steady proliferation of specialty and sub-specialty clinics so that it is not uncommon for a hospital to boast of 30 or more separate clinics meeting at different hours, five or six days a week. The chronically ill older patient who frequently suffers from several disease conditions, or poor families with several small children, are seen in several clinics which frequently meet on different days. Even if the clinical record is excellent and readily available, it is difficult if not impossible for any one physician to know the patient as a person and to coordinate his care.

Let the word go forth from this White House Conference on Health that America is prepared to assure all of its citizens equal access to health services as good as we can make them, and that the poor will no longer be forced to barter their dignity for their health.[18]

Although Dr. Yerby's comments are concerned mainly with services for the poor, the problem of fragmentation of professional service also applies to the more affluent—in not so acute a form, of course. The lessons learned from various group practices and prepayment plans had not been widely applied.

Under the auspices of the Children's Bureau of HEW, neighborhood based comprehensive care programs were being developed for infants and children. Because the mission of this agency is limited to children's programs, it did not seem feasible to sponsor centers caring for the entire family. It seemed likely that the children's comprehensive care programs would ultimately be integrated with new programs of family care developed under HEW auspices or with programs supported by the Office of Economic Opportunity.

In 1966 there appeared to be a consensus that health services for the poor were inadequate, when the President of the AMA, Dr. Charles L. Hudson, in his report to the House of Delegates (November 28, 1966) stated,

I propose that the A.M.A. and state and county medical societies launch a continuing program under predominantly private auspices to improve existing health care services and establish new services where they do not exist for all persons of whatever age, race, creed or color. I consider this kind of program a top priority A.M.A. obligation . . . I am not one who believes that pointing out the need is necessarily an indictment of our system of health care. I still believe it is excellent, but I trust you will agree that we are in a period of reassessment and realignment . . . I feel we have been over-occupied with constructing jurisdictional boundaries between the acknowledged private and public sectors of medical influence and activity.

And the Board of Trustees of the AMA received a report in 1966 (Report AA) from its Reference Committee on Insurance and Medical Service *B* recommending that the AMA offer to the Office of Economic Opportunity "the services of a technical advisory committee from the A.M.A. . . . pointing out that the lack of Association advice in the implementation of anti-poverty programs concerned with health could be to the detriment of both the programs and the future of American Medicine."

In June, 1966, the President's Consumer Advisory Council —a nonmedical group concerned with all aspects of consumer interest—published a report dealing with health services.[19] While acknowledging that of all purchases made, none is more difficult to judge than the quality of medical care, the report described the feelings of entitlement to health services which the consumer had developed. The report quoted President Johnson's statement that "we are learning to think of good health services, not as a privilege for the few, but as a basic right for all." It pointed to the increase in health expenditures from 4.5 percent of the gross national product in 1950 to 6 percent in 1964—a total expenditure of $36.8 billions in 1964.

Despite these expenditures, there remained millions of Americans who were receiving inferior health care and in some instances none at all. The Consumer Advisory Council report attributes these lacks to: (1) advances in medical knowledge that have outrun the supply of skilled personnel, (2) money spent on scientific research that has not been matched or even approached by funds to find better ways of delivering care, and (3) the number of people who can afford some medical care, but not as much as they need.

To deal with some of these problems, the report urged that efforts be made to stimulate prepayment group medical practices in contrast to traditional fee-for-service arrangements. It suggested the passage of legislation which would provide incentives in the form of loans and mortgages for doctors and dentists interested in developing such facilities and programs.

On "Meeting the Challenge of Family Practice" *

In the mid-1960's several reports concerned with the issue of educating physicians for family practice were submitted.** There were difficulties in arriving at a consensus on terminology: the National Commission on Community Health Services used the term "personal physicians"; the Citizens' Commission on Graduate Medical Education suggested "primary physician"; others suggested "general physician," in contrast to general practitioner. There seemed to be general agreement, that the concept of a general practitioner of years ago—that is, one who had responsibility for caring for all of man's ailments— was obsolete except for underdeveloped areas of the world. Each of these reports placed considerable emphasis on new educational programs for such new "generalist-specialists." Yet there had been rather substantial efforts to develop similar training programs in the past which interested virtually no trainees. One program was announced several years ago with much fanfare; it never had an applicant, although the director of the program was invited (to his embarrassment) to describe it as a "bold, new venture" at many meetings around the country. When there are repeated failures in spite of heroic efforts, it is perhaps appropriate to examine the social context in which the failures occur. The report of the Ad Hoc Committee on Education for Family Practice described the situation in this manner:

* Title of the Report of the Ad Hoc Committee on Education for Family Practice of the Council on Medical Education, American Medical Association, September, 1966.

** In addition to "Meeting the Challenge of Family Practice," the following reports appeared: The Coggeshall Report, "Planning for Medical Progress through Education," Association of American Medical Colleges, April, 1965; Report of the Citizens' Commission on Graduate Medical Education entitled "The Graduate Education of the Physician," American Medical Association, September, 1966; Report of the Task Force on Comprehensive Personal Health Services of the National Commission on Community Health Services entitled "Comprehensive Health Care: A Challenge to American Communities," May, 1966.

A Committee on Preparation for Family Practice (of the AMA) was appointed in 1957 and issued a report in 1959 which led to the establishment of new residency programs in family practice. Neither that report and the resultant training programs, nor other actions to date, most of which have been aimed at the area of graduate medical education, have yet been productive. The present Committee was therefore appointed to re-examine the problem and its causes and to suggest solutions which might be effective in increasing the supply of family physicians.

In order for training programs to emerge it would seem necessary for students to have an awareness of institutional contexts —or models—within which they may work with some degree of professional satisfaction and reward. The above report goes on to make these points:

The essential characteristics of a satisfactory model of family practice whether in a university medical center or a community hospital may be summarized as follows:

A full-time nucleus of family practice physicians, supplemented with part-time or voluntary staff, academically qualified and equivalent in quality and strength to other major clinical services.

An organizational unit within the teaching institution which provides voice and prerogatives equivalent to those of other specialties.

Control by the family practice staff of its clinical service.

Adequate facilities controlled by the family practice service within the teaching institution for the handling of ambulatory patients, hospitalized patients (both in the acute general hospital and in long-term institutions such as the nursing home) and for administration and research.

Arrangements for continuity of involvement and appropriate responsibility by the family practice service for patients transferred to other clinical services and institutions with the return of the patients to the family practice service at the appropriate time.

A defined population group consisting of families which represent a cross-section of the community, with the family practice service having the responsibility of providing or insuring comprehensive health care on a continuing basis.

Thus what was suggested more and more was a new institution which would perform the functions of a family physician. Whether the institution was defined as a "neighborhood health center," as in the antipoverty program, or "group practice" as in the report of the President's Consumer Advisory Council, is of little moment. There seemed to be consensus that it is increasingly difficult for the physician to provide adequate services as a solo practitioner. (This obviously does not mean that solo practice will decline precipitously—or that it should; the social changes under discussion will occur over decades although they may be catalyzed in a variety of ways.) But there is a "chicken and egg" problem here: do we first train the family practitioners or first establish the continuing, comprehensive community health centers? Because two decades of exhorting students to enter family practice have borne no fruit, empirically it would seem wise to set up the institutions which provide visible career opportunities. It may be that in this context the current generalist-specialists (pediatricians, internists, and obstetricians) working collaboratively may fill the need without a totally new program of training for family practitioners. If the institutional settings for practice develop, this problem will find a pragmatic —rather than a dogmatic—solution.

For all this to occur medicine must be oriented to the future as well as to its rich historical past. Let us therefore turn to the future.

4   Some Conceptual and Programmatic Issues

Facing Medicine

The Chinese Taoists conceive of a universe in which the yin, or female principle, battles endlessly with the yang, or male principle. Out of this interaction of forces a balance emerges which facilitates survival; the dominance of one or the other is attended by disability and decline in the organism. It is perhaps appropriate to speculate that various conceptual and institutional imbalances have developed in medicine—to its peril. The dominance of one set of forces over others may be predisposing us to problems which suggest some corrective measures. What may some of these be and what are their implications for programs?

Concepts of Health and Disease

Historically, medicine has been concerned with the understanding and management of disease. Certainly medical education and medical writings have been rooted in concepts of disease. Preventive efforts have also been rooted predominantly in disease prevention rather than health maintenance or conservation. Thus our knowledge of nutrition has increased and our nutritional programs have improved the health of our people as a consequence of our concern over nutritional-deficiency diseases. Such measures as the pasteurization of milk and the development of safe water supplies arose out of our concern over infectious diseases—as did the dramatic increase in our knowledge of immunology and its applications.

Although there is constant emphasis on the increasing complexity of medical services and their concomitant requirement for more personnel, it is well to note that increases in knowledge and its application over the past several decades has greatly saved physicians' time. The considerable decline, for example, in nutritional deficiency diseases, infectious diseases such as whooping cough, diphtheria, poliomyelitis, and measles—to mention but a few preventive efforts—indicates some of the conservation of manpower which has taken place. A literate mother today with adequate financial resources can feed her baby as effectively through her food selection in the supermarket as the pediatrician did three decades ago. Factors of this nature complicate planning for meeting our health manpower needs. Some of this reclaimed time may be going into the new Children's Bureau, Head Start, and Neighborhood Health Center programs, now that funds for professional services are available in these programs.

In recent years there has been a growing interest in health maintenance, in contrast to the traditional focus on disease and disease prevention. There are those in medicine who feel that this is an inappropriate emphasis which need not be a concern of physicians or that health maintenance will flow logically from a continuing emphasis on the study of the nature of disease. But such matters as the application of our newer knowledge of genetics in prevention, the role of family planning on health maintenance, developing early criteria for the prediction (and perhaps prevention) of disease, and the establishment of healthier environments (air, water, housing, and psychological and social environments) may be developed more fully in a non-hospital-, non-disease-oriented institutional context.

If an emphasis on the conservation of health develops, it need not displace the traditional emphasis on disease and its treatment, but new institutional forms and emphases will be required. If we are to move from a focus predominantly on pathology to a focus on pathogenesis and the preservation of social and biological effectiveness (health), the institutional base for research and services will need to shift in some degree from its hospital setting to a community health or outpatient program.

This is not an entirely new orientation; the epidemiologist has traditionally carried on his work by the study of populations in the community. We now need to apply the methods of the epidemiologist to the study of the evaluation and delivery of health services in the community as well as to disease and its prevention.

What are some of the developments which may be anticipated in a program of positive health services? The following are likely:

(1) The development of a new vocabulary of health analogous to a nosology for disease. It is interesting to note that medicine is so firmly rooted in disease concepts that we have virtually no terminology or classification for health. Particularly in relationship to social and psychological effectiveness, we have only the crudest kind of language—and no classification. Menninger has recognized this problem and has utilized such terms as "wellness," in contrast to sickness, and "weller-than-well," to describe a higher order of effectiveness.[1]

(2) Studies of the life histories and development of population groups in health rather than disease (longitudinal studies) —for which an outpatient institution is essential. There have been several such studies under pediatric and psychologic auspices over the past several decades.[2] In addition to adding to our knowledge of what keeps people well, such studies should be helpful in determining the antecedents—as well as the earliest manifestations—of disease. Indeed studies dynamically describing early deviations from health may make the current textbook descriptions of disease of historical interest. Such studies can also help us learn how people master adversity rather than succumb to it.

(3) The explorations of new techniques in early disease detection. The health manpower shortages, as well as favorable technological developments, suggest the application of newer techniques (particularly involving automation) in screening programs. Automation and the employment of nonprofessionals where feasible may permit scarce professional personnel to

devote their time to more complex problems. (Miller states that the *"future task of the well-trained will be to make it possible for less-trained people to perform adequately.* Professional development in this country should change. The professionals will not be primarily performing direct client service but making it possible for less trained people to perform such services." [3])
Automated techniques will also assist in developing quality control for screening programs. It is apparent that many biochemical screening techniques, electrocardiographic screening, recordings of blood pressure, and others, properly directed, lend themselves to such programs without sacrifice of quality. The proper utilization of computer programs will facilitate these developments. It is also apparent that much education—of professionals and the public—will be necessary for wide acceptance and application of such programs. Economic incentives for those attempting to keep people well will catalyze such developments. Prepayment health programs represent one such form of institutionalized economic incentive; but the field is largely uncharted and many explorations of new programs are in order. Certainly a balance must be struck between the desire for individual periodic examinations by the physician, and our personnel shortages for such services. With more sophisticated evaluation methods, we will have more objective data concerning the relative efficacy of these approaches in early disease detection.

The Medical Center and the Community Health Services

The traditional concerns of medicine with disease have made the hospital the major institutional focus of medicine. Hospital costs represent the largest single component of our health expenditures (see figure 3). There is a circularity in the continuation of the hospital as the primary medical institution; because it is the main institutional base (and most costly), it receives most attention, prestige, and financial support. And it remains the base of the health research enterprise. Its costliness requires more and more effort to revitalize it and to provide for its financing; and because it enjoys a central place in the health power structure, there is little effort to share the power and resources with other component health services. One of the major health programs in recent years, the Hill-Burton program, is a good example of the focus on hospital care, because it provides federal funds for hospital construction. On the other hand the Comprehensive Health Planning Act of 1965 will probably become a force to bring hospital and community health planning together.

Notes on the reinstitutionalization of hospital and community health services. The hospital as the major base of medical care has had an inhibitory effect on the development of community health services. The crisis in health services, especially in the big cities, has at last begun to direct attention to the long neglected problems of community health services. Although there are many people who assume that such services will develop best under the aegis of medical centers, with their traditional focus on hospital care, it is well to ponder whether this is the most effective way. The highest priority within the medical center hospital is, as it should be, on the care of the sick and hospitalized patient with a complex illness. In spite of many protests to the contrary, medical centers have not done a good job of providing continuing, comprehensive services for defined population groups; such services will inevitably have a lower priority in the value system of people charged with the care of patients suffering from complex, life-threatening illness.

It is suggested therefore that community health services be organized with autonomy and support which will make them attractive and intellectually stimulating settings in which to work. The lack of autonomy in such settings in the past (the outpatient departments of medical centers, or large public hospitals) has attracted relatively few talented, creative people, since the priority and prestige were always with the hospital-based program. Overlooked was the likelihood that the professional persons attracted to community health endeavors are somewhat different in talents, interests, and values from the hospital-oriented physician. Such people in the past found their major outlets in private practice which, satisfying though it may be for large numbers, does not provide institutional auspices for the development of teaching and research—or what the Ad Hoc Committee on Education for Family Practice refers to as a "model of family practice." Until these people are provided with institutional sponsorship in the community, it is unlikely that significant new developments will occur.

The above formulation of autonomy for community health services is predicated on a somewhat unorthodox view of health and hospital services (although it may be consistent with the ordering of services which may develop through the Regional Medical Program and the Comprehensive Health Planning and Public Health Services Amendments of 1966—P.L. 89–749 and its Partnership for Health Amendments of 1967). Rather than speaking of hospital services and community health services, it is probably more effective to conceive of (1) *medical center services,* in which the medical center hospital cares for patients with complex illness and its outpatient service serves as a diagnostic consultation resource, the Mayo clinic model—a function that is generally discharged well in university as well as nonuniversity medical centers; the failure to differentiate this function from that of continuing, comprehensive, family care often obscures perception of how inadequately these family care outpatient services are generally provided for poor families; and (2) *community health services* in which the doctor's office and/or clinic is linked with a community hospital in order to care for families comprehensively. Thus the doctor's office and community hospital are viewed as an institution, with a relationship to the medical center services which does not duplicate or rival those services (a pattern which is costly and often ineffective). These relationships are illustrated diagrammatically as in figure 8.

Medical Center
with focus on disease;
episodic care

Community Health Services
with focus on prevention
and continuing,
comprehensive family care

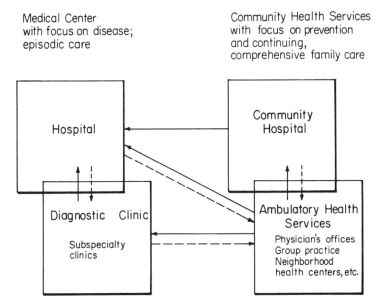

Fig. 8. Suggested relation of community health services to the medical center. Solid arrows indicate referral of sick patients; broken arrows indicate referral of discharged patients.

Notes on hospital financing. The basis for financing hospital care merits serious reevaluation, because hospitals are in continuing—and increasing—financial crisis. The financing of hospital care, through private and public funds, is dependent upon a per diem rate for each patient. Thus there is a premium placed on keeping all hospital beds filled, as any practicing physician learns if the bed occupancy of his hospital drops off.

Although technically difficult to work out, some system of economic incentives for reducing bed occupancy (without doing an injustice to patient care, of course) should be considered. For example, more ready access to diagnostic services without hospitalization (often rendered difficult under existing insurance plans), more adequate home health services and homemaker services, as well as a better distribution between hospital and nursing home and other less costly services, might considerably reduce the need for hospitalization. But this may not happen if there is a continuing financial need to keep hospital beds filled. Small wonder that it becomes difficult to define how many hospital beds a community needs! One study indicated that while the ratio of beds to population in an area sets a top limit on hospital utilization, more subtly the bed supply also influences the lower limit. Thus, given insurance, available beds tend to be used.[4] The same factors operate in publicly sponsored hospital programs, because these hospital budgets also are generally based on per diem rates. It is extremely difficult, short of financial crisis, to eliminate beds or hospitals in any community. Regional hospital planning councils (or area health planning groups under the Comprehensive Health Planning Act) will experience more community pressure to withhold support for adding beds and expensive equipment without demonstrating need. These councils will also move toward reorganization, especially for pediatric and maternity beds which are not usable for other purposes and which commonly are severely underutilized.[5] Incentives for the development of better cost accounting will be introduced to determine better distribution of costs.

The Medicare legislation places some pressures on communities, and provides some economic incentives, for developing a broader spectrum of services, such as nursing home facilities and home visits by nurses and other health workers, in addition to the more costly hospital services. Since the legislation provides only for patients over sixty-five years of age, this may not be a sufficiently potent force to stimulate the development of new institutional arrangements in communities. The Medicare regulation stipulating that utilization review committees evaluate the necessity for extended hospitalization is a step toward a conservation of hospital beds and funds. The difficulties of such evaluations are many, and it remains to be seen whether this process becomes perfunctory or whether it stimulates a more critical review of the utilization of hospital and other community health resources. One of the great difficulties in any such effort is the matter of developing quality control in the area of professional services. The possibilities of unfortunate bureaucratic controls developing are real, but, with rising costs and the pressures for accurate accounting and cost analysis, pragmatic solutions will develop. The Medicare legislation, combined with other developments such as the growth of prepayment health programs (which include hospitalization costs), may result in much more effort being directed toward planning for a spectrum of community health services which permit medical care programs to be tailored to the unique needs of the patient (often referred to as progressive patient care). It is obvious that when a spectrum of services is not available, the most costly service—hospitalization—will be utilized extensively.

If economic incentives for hospitalization were removed (or conversely, if there were economic penalties for inappropriate hospitalization—however difficult this is to define), we might see the emergence of more vigorous and imaginative preventive programs. For example, since approximately 12 percent of short-stay general hospital beds are occupied by patients as a result of accidents, hospitals might develop a vested interest in accident prevention. It is small wonder that some of the most effective materials on accident prevention have been developed by insurance companies.

Another example of possible excessive utilization is the matter of tonsilectomy and adenoidectomy. The National Health Survey has reported that 1,063,000 such operations are performed each year. This figure represents approximately 9 percent of all surgical operations in general, short-stay hospitals. Since these operations are not commonly indicated, one may wonder whether they would be performed less frequently if there were economic gains in the nonperformance. Obviously a prepayment health program would have much to gain financially from fewer nonessential operations—to say nothing of reducing the hazards resulting from the procedure (it is estimated that in the United States 139 deaths per year result from complications of these operations).

Notes on hospital management. The controversial matter of management must concern anyone interested in hospital costs. There is much debate about whether rising costs result in part as a consequence of inefficient management. Some of the rising costs are due to the gradual rise in the level of compensation of hospital employees, which were at ridiculously low levels during the depression years. The personnel crisis in hospitals has resulted in an economic catching up process, but a cultural lag has developed. Because of the image that hospitals have developed as undesirable places in which to work, the recruitment of nonprofessionals of ability has been difficult. At the professional level the recruitment of nurses is a significant national problem, because the low salaries are not at all commensurate with the educational and training background required.

Modern management methods have been slow in coming to hospitals. The nonprofit nature of most hospitals has probably obscured responsibility, since the community in one way or another must meet the costs—whatever these may be. Business organizations compete more aggressively for managerial talent, and it may well be that the field of hospital administration has been at a disadvantage in recruitment. The nonprofit nature of hospital corporations precludes providing some of the economic benefits to hospital administrators which are available to business executives. Certainly there has been all too little attention given to the recruitment, education, and training of hospital management personnel. There are at the present time 24 university schools of hospital administration in the United States (of which 16 are members of the Association of University Programs in Hospital Administration) graduating approximately 350 students per year. For an industry which is charged with the expenditures of approximately $15 billion per year, this is hardly adequate, especially because these graduates are employed in a wide variety of health administrative services—in addition to being employed in the 7,000 hospitals in the United States.

A largely unexplored pattern for improving the effectiveness and innovative capacities of hospital management, while perhaps enhancing the recruitment potentialities, might be the development of management corporations which would, on a contractual basis, administer the voluntary and public hospitals. Thus community responsibility for the corporate ownership of the hospital could be maintained, while introducing considerable flexibility in administrative patterns based on the development of wholesome competition among the management corporations. Management groups could provide greater degrees of management specialization and subspecialization than individual hospitals can under present arrangements. These management firms could also provide more significant challenges as well as economic incentives for executives, which could be equivalent to those of large corporations. A similar arrangement has been employed in such programs as the Job Corps of the Office of Economic Opportunity. Several large corporations, on contract with this federal agency, are the administrators of the programs. Although this was a novel venture, the management groups proved remarkably adept at mobilizing resources for the development of very complex programs. Hospital management has its unique complexities, particularly because of the role of the medical staff, which has much authority but relatively little operational responsibility. These problems are not insoluble however as is evidenced by the contracting of such services as laundry, food, parking, and computer utilization to private firms by many hospitals—services which traditionally have been performed directly by the hospital.

Medicine and Society

The increasing knowledge available to us has had far reaching effects on our society. The average life span increased by ten years from 1937 to 1964, to an average age of seventy years. This change has come about not only because of increasing medical knowledge, but also because of generally improved living conditions. But we may question, at this stage in our development, whether we are now keeping pace with our potentialities for the conservation of life. Population growth, population mobility (with increasing urbanization and suburbanization), accentuation of poverty in the midst of plenty, and rapid technological progress, which introduces hazards (air and water pollution and potential noise and radiation trauma) while also improving our environment, are factors to which we have not made an effective accommodation.

The application of our knowledge to improving medical services alone, while important and humane, will not result in major improvements in our health record. What is needed now is a partnership between medicine and society for the application of what we know. A few examples may illustrate the potential results of this partnership:

(1) If we are to conserve life, the prevention of accidents (now the leading cause of death among children and the fourth most common cause for all age groups) must become a more serious and effective endeavor. Although the health professions deal with the end results of accidents (injuries) and can help to dramatize the problem, the development of effective measures for prevention is a *social* problem. Dealing with the problem obviously involves such complex processes as city planning, road building, and automobile design, as well as education. To develop preventive programs and measures, resources and talent must be made available. To do this we need some process by which priorities may be established, incentives developed, and resultant programs pursued.

(2) The results of environmental pollution become medical problems, but prevention of noise and radiation contamination and air and water pollution are the responsibility of society as a whole. The widespread use of pesticides and drugs poses unique problems. Because of a lack of consistent planning, these problems gradually creep up on us, and it is not until a major crisis develops (as in periods of severe air contamination over our large cities or severe water shortages or obvious water contamination) that we are moved to act. Medical knowledge, along

with other scientific advances, can contribute to planning, but society as a whole must act and provide appropriate resources.

(3) Although we know much about prevention, we do not know all that we would like to know about preventing cancer and cardiovascular disease. As additional research is carried on, educational service programs can do much to minimize hazards. This is a social problem of course involving education in the role of exercise and diet in preventing cardiovascular disease and the hazards of smoking. The employment of our educational resources in these efforts has only begun. The regional medical programs on heart disease, cancer, stroke, and related diseases are an institutional approach to these problems on a national basis.

(4) Psychiatric disorders have been characterized as the nation's greatest health problem; psychiatric services account for 50 percent of our hospitalized patients. Perhaps no group of disorders is as inextricably interwoven with the quality of living. Since the life situation of the person is so significant in the development of psychiatric disorders, the very definition of psychiatric concerns becomes difficult. The emerging programs for comprehensive community mental health services tend to reflect the broad, ecological view; this contrasts with the concern of some clinicians that psychiatry confine its activities to more formally organized individual and group psychiatric treatment. Considerable conceptual clarification is desirable in order to develop programs of greater specificity; out of such clarification more adequate social action may result.

(5) One of our most serious losses of human potentialities occurs among children as a consequence of impoverished environmental circumstances. This problem is detailed in the report of the Planning Committee for Project Head Start of the Office of Economic Opportunity.

There is considerable evidence that the early years of childhood are the most critical point in the poverty cycle. During these years the creation of learning patterns, emotional development and the formation of individual expectations and aspirations take place at a very rapid pace. For the child of poverty there are clearly observable deficiencies in the processes which lay the foundation for a pattern of failure—and thus a pattern of poverty—throughout the child's entire life.

Within recent years there has been experimentation and research designed to improve opportunities for the child of poverty. While much of this work is not yet complete there is adequate evidence to support the view that special programs can be devised for these four and five year olds which will improve both the child's opportunities and achievements.

It is clear that successful programs of this type must be comprehensive, involving activities generally associated with the fields of health, social services, and education. Similarly it is clear that the program must focus on the problems of child and parent and that these activities need to be carefully integrated with programs for the school years . . . The Office of Economic Opportunity should generally avoid financing programs which do not have at least a minimum level and quality of activities from each of the three fields of effort.

The need for and urgency of these programs is such that they should be initiated immediately.[6]

Although an ultimate solution is the elimination of poverty and its depriving circumstances (many of these children are growing up in families of second- and third-generation poverty), it seems desirable to provide some institutional assistance in the form of day care and early childhood educational programs, along with more effective elementary school programs to enhance the developmental capacities of these children, physically, socially, emotionally, and culturally.[7] Again, this is not an exclusively medical problem; all of society has a stake in it.

(6) We have now dropped to sixteenth among the countries of the world in our infant mortality record. Repeated studies of our population monotonously reveal that the major contributing factor is the high mortality rate in the nonwhite, poor population. Although greater provision and utilization of prenatal health services would probably contribute to a reduction in this

rate, it is also reasonable to assume that poverty is a major factor. Thus, our medical knowledge may be helpful, but improving living conditions through better incomes, housing, nutrition, family planning, and reduction of social and emotional stress is perhaps more significant.

(7) Our medical knowledge enables us to immunize against a number of diseases. Yet all too few children and adults receive the benefits. Again this is not a medical problem; it is one of health education and social application of what we know. As our knowledge of the pathogenesis of disease improves, we may anticipate the introduction of many other preventive measures —in psychological and social, as well as in physical, development.

The first two-thirds of the twentieth century have been characterized by significant and constructive advances in the field of health. In education for the health professions, further advances will depend upon greater flexibility in the educational process in the light of constant improvements in preprofessional education. Such flexibility will be made possible by increasing sophistication in the evaluation of the performance of professional work rather than predominantly in the teaching of content.[8,9]

With innovations in medical education and education for other health professions under way, a reinstitutionalization of education is taking place. Few of the innovations are of the significance of the introduction of the clinical clerkship and the teaching of the sciences basic to medicine at the turn of the century and the interdepartmental committee approach to teaching introduced at Western Reserve Medical School in 1952; it may be inevitable, as a result of the increasing complexity of the educational process, that the next steps will come more slowly and be less dramatic.

Increasing qualitative and quantitative demands face education for all the health professions. Recent publications indicate the difficulties in defining the precise needs for personnel in the health professions.[10,11] There seems to be consensus that our affluent society can absorb sizable increases in our output of health personnel. The establishment of new schools will of course contribute to the output, but earlier increases will be effected by expansion of existing programs. Although there is always anxiety concerning the dilution of the quality of education with expansion, there is no evidence that any group desires any deterioration in quality. The challenge is to continue attempting to meet needs without sacrificing quality.

There is consensus that aides and assistants for the health professional will play a more important role in the provision of health services in the future. Education for the health professions will need to incorporate preparation for supervisory responsibilities while exploring the feasibility of new kinds of assistance; any effort to stretch the time and effort of professional persons is very much in order.

The research advances of recent decades have generated significant public support. Although there is some conjecture that advances in research in the health sciences have not been communicated adequately to the public, the increasing expectations by the public would belie this.[12] What may be needed is greater public sophistication concerning the significance of basic research and the complexities of transferring research findings to services. A recent report to the President on the Research Programs of the National Institutes of Health states the issue as follows: "The continued advancement of fundamental research is essential as the base for the qualitative and quantitative expansion of the educational process and to enlarge the body of knowledge from which practical results can be derived." [13] Public expectations need not lead to an either-or approach—that is, support for either research or services. An affluent society can afford both. New institutional approaches to the organization and support of research programs may be anticipated because of the increase in their magnitude.[14]

In health services some delay in translating new knowledge into programs may result from the relative lack of an institutional form well known to industry—that of product development. Clinical programs in and out of universities tend to take on this function, but it occurs slowly and generally without very much support, with the exception of new knowledge in the drug industry where the product is more easily defined.

The rising expectations for more and better health services will continue to stimulate new approaches to the financing and delivery of these services. In addition to traditional fee-for-service arrangements, comprehensive prepayment plans, insurance-indemnity programs, and new publicly financed programs will be explored. Various models merit testing; most of these combine old and emerging patterns of care. Kerr White suggests that the prototype for health-service systems is a public utility model—that of the airlines. He goes on to indicate that "such a model . . . is in keeping with the best traditions of this country in its mix of public and private financing, participation and control: it encourages innovation and experimentation and is based on the most constructive aspects of human motivation and competition." [15] That physicians are willing to participate in the reorganization of services which has been going on is evidenced in part by the gradual decline in the percentage of those engaged in individual practice. That they and others in the health professions are interested in improving the quality of health services to the poor is apparent in their participation in neighborhood health centers and other health programs.

Since every new program is subject to the query "Does it provide better care?" there will be more effort to measure quality of service—a process which has seemed impossible to professional persons in the past. The literature reveals much interest, but little competence, at present.[16] How to measure quality is a crucial matter for study, because there is consensus that total expenditure alone is not a true measure of the quality of health services.

The complexity of the national health enterprise has reached a point at which a national strategy is desirable. Consideration of issues relating to health is the concern of every department and agency of government. The relevance for health of programs in the Departments of Agriculture, Housing and Urban Development, and Labor, in addition to Health, Education and Welfare is apparent. The State Department, concerned with atomic energy and international health, also has significant health interests. It would seem appropriate therefore that a Presidential Council of Health Advisors, somewhat analogous to the Council of Economic Advisors, be established to develop and pursue the strategy. The tactical approach would remain with individual public agencies, voluntary agencies, the professions, and the public through their choices among alternatives.

In 1967 the National Academy of Sciences moved to form a new Board of Medicine in response to the "growing concern on the part of the Academy, members of the medical profession, and a number of Federal agencies as to how our rapidly expanding biomedical knowledge can be more effectively applied in response to critical human needs." Its directive is to identify "urgent problems, to be imaginative in seeking solutions, and innovative in recommending public policy." The Board will report directly to the Council of the National Academy of Sciences. This new group has the potential for developing policy and strategy for a national health program. It could complement any agency which develops for the planning and coordination of intragovernmental health programs.

The growth of our society and its increasing complexity demands new approaches. One of our leaders in higher education, Chancellor Samuel Gould of the State University of New York, has defined the challenge as follows:

Our present methods of responding to the changing needs of the world are more closely characterized as a patchwork approach, rather than one of bold and inventive planning. With all the ingredients present to tell us what the world has in store, we are still adapting old methods and making minor revisions and emergency moves; we are still desperately trying to pour new wine into old bottles instead of recognizing that the new vintages may require quite different sorts of receptacles . . .

We patch here and there, but we still procrastinate about meeting the issues squarely. Only now, years later than it should have happened, do we see a general stirring, a growing sense of urgency among educational leaders regarding the need for clearly establishing the philosophy of their institutions and systematically planning their long-range futures. Only now is there an increasing awareness that, given the rapidly changing world we live in, we can no longer expect anything to remain the same, even educational anythings.[17]

5 Approaches

to Complexity

Lest any impression be left with the reader that our health problems have simple or unitary solutions, a few additional notes are in order. For the complexity of health programs, like all complex institutions, renders it inevitable that the manipulation of one factor influences all the others. This is not to suggest that we forego change because of its complexity. Instead it is desirable to have a strategy for change based on a concept of the processes of health and disease along with an understanding of the methodological and technical advances that are taking place. We have attempted to illustrate this complexity through a series of diagrams which may be helpful to the reader and which may elaborate some of the concepts of the preceding text.

It is a truism that tasks in the health professions have increased in number and complexity. In the early decades of this century for example the objective of medical education was monolithic: the preparation of general physicians. Over the past four decades a much more complex range of opportunities and objectives has faced the student and medical education.[1] These changes are the products of advances in our medical knowledge and technology, as well as sociologic changes associated with rising standards of living, urbanization and suburbanization, better transportation, and shifting institutional patterns in medical practice—particularly group practice and the increasing involvement of university medical centers in patient care.

In the face of mounting specialization, the job of the health worker remains substantially the same—evaluating the functional capacity of the individual.[2] The integration of the many factors acting upon the organism from within and without is the most difficult task in health education. Alan Gregg epitomized this problem in a discussion of multiple causes of disease as follows:

Almost by definition an organism is an association of organs so intimately related that no part can be changed without changing in some way and in some measure all the others . . . It is intellectual weakness that prompts us to ascribe a given result to only one sufficient cause. We ignore the value of suspecting that a result may be due to a convergence of several "causes" which separately or in some other sequence will not produce the result we seek to explain. This tendency to overlook convergent or multiple causation seduces us as an unrecognized temptation in our enthusiasm as teachers to make things "clear".[3]

To illustrate the conceptual complexity, we have developed the diagrammatic scheme shown in figure 9.[4]

This approach permits a visualization of the interaction of the internal environment (biologic factors) with the physical environment (including social factors) and the emotional environment (the psychological life history) and their combined impact on the functional or homeostatic capacity of the person. This scheme can be used to evaluate functional capacity, seen (by the observer) in quantitative terms, by assigning significance to the surface area of the central circle or amoeboid pattern. Thus, by a series of diagrams over time, the changing pattern of adaptation may be illustrated. The diagrammatic scheme for a child with bronchial asthma (figure 10) shows considerable change in functional capacity over even short periods of time.

Undoubtedly the judgment concerning the functional capacity of any person is influenced by the background, education, and experience of the observer. To illustrate the interaction of these factors in determining the capacity of the student physician for making such judgments we have suggested a model (figure 11) similar to those just discussed.

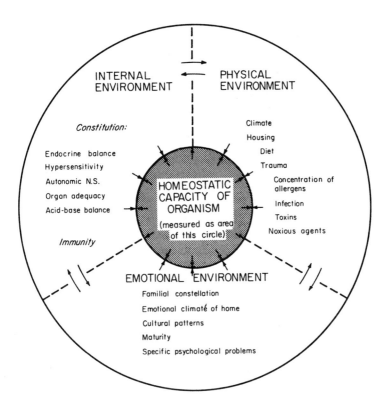

Fig. 9. A conceptual model illustrating, in part, the interacting factors basic for an understanding of the patient. Helping the student to conceptualize this interaction is one of the challenges to clinical training.
SOURCE: J. B. Richmond and S. L. Lustman, "Total Health: A Conceptual Visual Aid," *J. Med. Educ. 29*:23 (1954).

Figure 11 does not account for the experience and additional educational background the physician acquires through his years of practice. The deficiencies of continuing education for the physician have been dealt with elsewhere. It may well be

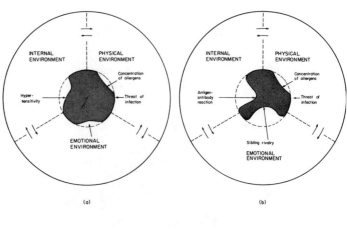

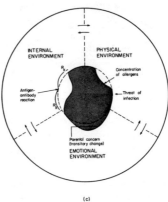

Fig. 10. A diagrammatic representation of some of the factors influencing an "asthmatic" child: (a) marginal adjustment; (b) an emotional crisis, centering about sibling rivalry, triggers an asthmatic attack (antigen-antibody reaction may be dominant factor on another occasion); (c) return to marginal adjustment with pharmacologic and psychologic therapy.

SOURCE: J. B. Richmond and S. L. Lustman, "Total Health: A Conceptual Visual Aid," *J. Med. Educ.* 29:23 (1954).

that the regional medical programs now developing will provide for the first time adequate resources and settings for a more effective program of continuing education for physicians. They certainly offer the potential for basing the educational program around the physician's daily problems in patient care.

If medical education is to fulfill its obligations to society, it should adapt to several changes now taking place. Among these changes are the following:

(1) The improved educational background of medical students today. Since the launching of Sputnik I, there has been a decided emphasis on educational achievement, which reaches into the elementary and high schools and continues through collegiate education. As a consequence, entering medical students today have often gained considerable background in the subject matter of the first two years of medical school. It has been suggested in a recent paper by Lowell Coggeshall that this trend will continue.[5] It would seem in order therefore to liberalize the medical school curriculum and to permit many more alternatives than has been conventional. Paul Sanazaro sees the following trend developing: "the medical school may well evolve into a college, comparable to colleges in the university. In place of the fixed medical curriculum, we see the emergence of multiple majors within medicine. Each department within the college becomes, in essence, a school offering courses at the undergraduate and graduate levels. Some of these would be required of all candidates for the M.D. degree. Others would be offered for special students or for selected majors. The number and types of majors offered by a medical college would depend on the college's educational goals and resources." [6]

(2) The increasing period of postgraduate training. Since almost all students now go on to specialty training (even for family practice) for from three to five years after graduation from medical school, it seems inappropriate to attempt to be encyclopedic in curriculum content—a course of action that was justified when the four year medical school experience was the terminal education of the physician.

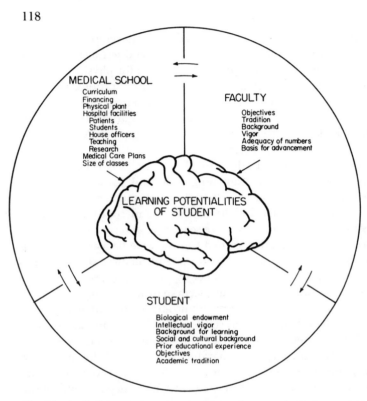

Fig. 11. A diagrammatic representation of some of the factors influencing the learning potentialities of the student.
SOURCE: J. B. Richmond, "Report of the First Institute on Clinical Teaching." Report of the Sixth Teaching Institute of the Association of American Medical Colleges, Swampscott, Mass., Oct. 7–11, 1958.

(3) The tremendous increase in knowledge. The problem of teaching what we know is being dealt with in part by an earlier introduction of programs in human biology in the elementary, high school, and college curricula. The tendency therefore to expand the medical school curriculum by accretion does not seem rational. Indeed Robert Oppenheimer has suggested that increasing scientific knowledge might simplify the teaching

process in some ways. He observes, "On the other hand, there is a more encouraging aspect of this scientific knowledge. As it grows, things, in some ways, get much simpler. They do not get simpler because one discovers a few fundamental principles which the man in the street can understand and from which he can derive everything else. But we do find an enormous amount of order. The world is not random and whatever order it has seems in large part 'fit,' as Thomas Jefferson said, for the human intelligence. The enormous variety of facts yields to some kind of arrangement, simplicity, generalization." [7]

During the postwar period medical educators have been endeavoring to deal with these problems by liberalization of the educational process. Some have done this by reordering the content of the curriculum and placing the responsibility for teaching in faculty committees somewhat outside the usual departmental structure (the approach of Western Reserve Medical School in Cleveland); others have increased the opportunities for research; still others have tended to provide options to the student for shortening or lengthening the medical school years. Perhaps the pervasive trend has been to individualize the student's program, largely by providing him with an opportunity to exercise options on how he is to use his time.

(4) The rapid expansion of research. Medical research in the United States has been developed largely in university medical centers, in contrast to many other countries in which research institutes carry on this work. The research orientation of the medical schools offers many opportunities for medical students and other health workers. It also adds to the institutional complexity and offers a challenge for effective institutional organization.

(5) The expansion of patient care. In the developing complex of health services, the university medical centers are at the hub. They have the responsibility for developing models of excellence for the care of individual patients. As Dean Ebert of the Harvard Medical School suggests,

Medical schools must move beyond their current fragmented efforts in health care and become involved in solving the problem of providing total care for a community or population . . .

In order to execute these illustrative programs, it is evident that a variety of skills will be needed. Clinical facilities must be involved, not in a peripheral way, but with major commitment; and they must learn to work directly with people in public health (or preventive medicine) as well as with economists, sociologists, and other social scientists.

Efforts to plan for health care will be of little value if the models developed remain encapsulated within the university. The medical schools cannot and should not attempt to provide all the care in a community, but they should develop models which can be replicated. They should also participate with communities willing to experiment with new models.[8]

How to provide demonstrations in the delivery of health services without impairing the research and teaching functions of the medical center remains a central challenge for medical education.

Perhaps no problem facing the health professions today is more complex than that of manpower.[9,10] In planning for meeting our needs, it is apparent that the manipulation of any one factor influences all others. We have attempted to illustrate the relationships among a few of the factors affecting the quality, quantity, and distribution of resources (figure 12).

Although the medical schools have increased the number of graduates from 5,097 in 1940 to 7,409 in 1965, we also certified 1,488 physicians from abroad in 1965 (a five-fold increase over 1950). Thus we have an unfavorable "balance of trade" currently, importing rather than exporting, and in the process depleting the physician resources of many underdeveloped countries. It is estimated that we have a shortage of 125,000 practicing nurses. There are no easy answers to these complex problems. Shall we educate and train more of each, or shall we develop new health workers to take over some of the work traditionally assigned to these groups? Or may the redeployment

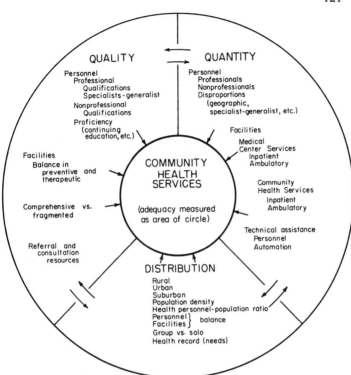

Fig. 12. Dynamics of health manpower resources.

and redistribution of health workers enhance their productivity and render estimates of shortages obsolete? How much responsibility can we turn over to nonmedical personnel for work on environmental sanitation? And how much professional time can we conserve by placing more responsibility for such things as nutrition and immunization in the hands of an increasingly literate, informed, and health-oriented population?

Judgments must be made and a program for social action implemented, just as the clinician arrives at a prescription for management. More and better data derived from demonstration, research, and evaluation will improve our capacities for making judgments in public planning and policy formation. But data will never be complete, and we will never be relieved of the responsibility for decision making, just as in the management of the individual patient we never have all the data we wish. Nevertheless we can revise our plans and programs in the light of new data and new developments.

Thus, although our problems are complex, our approaches to complexity need not lead to inertia. Our informed, nonmedical colleagues have the expectation that we can develop systematic approaches to problem solving in the field of health. Elinor Langer makes the point cogently:

I think the policy-makers are burdened by what they perceive as the enormous intellectual complexity of the task. Medical ideologists, as well as medical idealists, seem to have passed out of currency in this country, and the men now making decisions are, if anything, too modest and too humble. They number among themselves—and they certainly have access to—the best informed authorities on medical services in America and abroad. They have a clear perception of what the problems are. But they say they don't know what the answers are, or how the problems can be solved, or what they ought to do next. They are afraid of imposing overall or systematic solutions, partly because they are afraid their solutions might be wrong ones, partly because they begin with a bias against systematic solutions in general. Instead they try to do a little bit of everything at once.[11]

References

Chapter 1. The Educational Revolution
and the Guild Establishment
(1900–1940)

1. Flexner, A. *Medical Education in the United States and Canada.* The Carnegie Foundation for the Advancement of Teaching, Bulletin No. 4. New York, 1910.

2. Flexner, A. *Medical Education: A Comparative Study.* New York: Macmillan, 1925.

3. "A New Departure in Medical Education (Editorial)." *New Eng. J. Med. 275:*1020 (1966).

4. Freymann, J. G. "Leadership in American Medicine: A Matter of Personal Responsibility." *New Eng. J. Med. 270:*710 (1964).

5. Fishbein, M. *A History of the American Medical Association 1847–1947: With the Biographies of the Presidents of the Association by Walter A. Bierring: And with Histories of the Publications, Councils, Bureaus, and Other Official Bodies.* Philadelphia: Saunders, 1947.

6. *National Health Survey 1935–36, Preliminary Reports. The Magnitude of the Chronic Disease Problem in the United States.* Sickness and Medical Care Series, Bull. 6, NIH, USPHS, Washington, 1938.

7. *Report on Medical Manpower by the Board of Trustees to the House of Delegates of the A.M.A.,* Annual Meeting June 18–22, 1967, Atlantic City, New Jersey.

8. Gilb, C. L. *Hidden Hierarchies: The Professions and Government.* New York: Harper & Row, 1966.

9. *Medical Care for the American People: The Final Report of the Committee on the Costs of Medical Care,* adopted October 31, 1932. The University of Chicago Press, 1932.

10. "The Advancement of Knowledge for the Nation's Health." A Report to the President on the Research Programs of the National

Institutes of Health. U. S. Dept. of Health, Education and Welfare, PHS, 1967.

11. *American Medicine: Expert Testimony Out of Court.* 2 vols. New York: The American Foundation, 1937.

12. "The Committee of Physicians for the Presentation of Certain Principles and Proposals in the Provision of Medical Care." *New Eng. J. Med. 217:*798 (November 1937).

13. "Editorial, The American Foundation Proposals for Medical Care." *JAMA 109:*1281 (Oct. 16, 1937)

14. Sigerist, H. E. *The University at the Crossroads.* New York: Henry Schuman, 1946.

15. "The Graduate Education of Physicians." The Report of the Citizens' Commission on Graduate Medical Education. Chicago: AMA, 1966.

16. Somers, A., "Conflict, Accommodation, and Progress: Some Socioeconomic Observations on Medical Education and the Practicing Profession," in *Medical Education and Medical Care: Interactions and Prospects.* Evanston, Illinois: AAMC, 1961.

Chapter 2. The Scientific Revolution and the Academic Establishment (1940–1960)

1. Weinberg, Alvin M., cited in "Biomedical Policy: LBJ's Query Leads to an Illuminating Conference." *Science 154:*619 (Nov. 4, 1966).

2. Drew, E. B. "The Health Syndicate: Washington's Noble Conspirators." *The Atlantic 220:*75 (December 1967).

3. Hanft, R. "National Health Expenditures, 1950–65." *Social Security Bulletin 30:*3 (February 1967).

4. "Research and Medical Education." Report of the Ninth Teaching Institute of the Association of American Medical Colleges. ed. Julius H. Comroe, Jr. Colorado Springs, Colorado, Dec. 3–7, 1961.

5. "Report of the First Institute on Medical School Administration." Report of the Eleventh Teaching Institute of the Association of American Medical Colleges. ed. Robert M. Bucher and Lee Powers. Atlanta, Georgia, Oct. 5–8, 1963.

6. "Medical Education and Practice: Relationships in a Changing Society." Report of the Tenth Teaching Institute of the Association of American Medical Colleges. ed. Stewart G. Wolf, Jr. and Ward Darley. Colorado Springs, Colorado, Dec. 9–12, 1962.

7. Kerr, C. *The Uses of the University.* Cambridge, Mass.: Harvard University Press, 1963.

8. Perkins, J. A. *The University in Transition.* Princeton, N. J.: Princeton University Press, 1966.

9. "Medical Ventures and the University: New Values and New Validities." Report of the Thirteenth Teaching Institute of the Association of American Medical Colleges, Third Institute on Administration. ed. Douglas M. Knight and E. Shepley Nourse. Bal Harbour, Florida, Dec. 12–15, 1965.

10. Carroll, A. J. *A Study of Medical College Costs.* Evanston, Illinois: AAMC, 1958.

11. Carroll, A. J., and W. Darley. "Medical College Costs." *J. Med. Educ. 42*:1 (January 1967).

12. Russell, J. M. *1963–64 Annual Report of the John and Mary R. Markle Foundation* (522 Fifth Avenue, N. Y.), pp. 12, 13.

13. *Bulletin of the Association of American Medical Colleges 1*:3 (Aug. 17, 1966).

14. Greenberg, D. S. "LBJ Directive: He Says Spread the Research Money." *Science 149*:1483 (Sept. 24, 1965).

15. Pake, G. "Basic Research and Financial Crisis in the Universities." *Science 157*:517 (Aug. 4, 1967).

16. Carey, W. D., cited in "Biomedical Policy: LBJ's Query Leads to an Illuminating Conference." *Science 154*:618 (Nov. 4, 1966).

17. Jencks, C. "A New Breed of BA's: Some Alternatives to Boredom and Unrest." *New Republic 153*:17 (Oct. 25, 1965).

18. *Datagram 7,* No. 5. Evanston, Illinois: AAMC, November, 1965.

19. Walsh, J. "NIH: Demand Increases for Applications of Research." *Science 153*:149 (July 8, 1966).

20. Russell, J. M., *1965–66 Annual Report of the John and Mary R. Markle Foundation* (522 Fifth Avenue, N. Y.), pp. 8, 9.

21. Coggeshall, L. T. "Planning for Medical Progress Through Education." A Report Submitted to the Executive Council of the Association of American Medical Colleges. April, 1965.

22. "The Teaching of Physiology, Biochemistry, Pharmacology." Report of the First Teaching Institute of the Association of American Medical Colleges. Atlantic City, N. J., Oct. 19–23, 1953.

"The Teaching of Pathology, Microbiology, Immunology, Genetics." Report of the Second Teaching Institute of the Association of American Medical Colleges. French Lick, Ind., Oct. 10–15, 1954.

"The Teaching of Anatomy and Anthropology in Medical Education." Report of the Third Teaching Institute of the Association of

American Medical Colleges. Swampscott, Mass., Oct. 18–22, 1955.

"The Appraisal of Applicants to Medical Schools." Report of the Fourth Teaching Institute of the Association of American Medical Colleges. Colorado Springs, Colo., Nov. 7–10, 1956.

"The Ecology of the Medical Student." Report of the Fifth Teaching Institute of the Association of American Medical Colleges. Atlantic City, N. J., Oct. 15–19, 1957.

"Report of the First Institute on Clinical Teaching." Report of the Sixth Teaching Institute of the Association of American Medical Colleges. Swampscott, Mass., Oct. 7–11, 1958.

"Report of the Second Institute on Clinical Teaching." Report of the Seventh Teaching Institute of the Association of American Medical Colleges. Chicago, Ill., Oct. 27–31, 1959.

"Medical Education and Medical Care: Interactions and Prospects." Report of the Eighth Teaching Institute of the Association of American Medical Colleges. Hollywood Beach, Fla., Nov. 1–3, 1960.

"Research and Medical Education." Report of the Ninth Teaching Institute of the Association of American Medical Colleges. ed. Julius H. Comroe, Jr. Colorado Springs, Colo., Dec. 3–7, 1961.

"Medical Education and Practice: Relationships and Responsibilities in a Changing Society." Report of the Tenth Teaching Institute of the Association of American Medical Colleges. ed. Stewart G. Wolf, Jr. and Ward Darley. Colorado Springs, Colo., Dec. 9–12, 1962.

"Report of the First Institute on Medical School Administration." Report of the Eleventh Teaching Institute of the Association of American Medical Colleges. ed. Robert M. Bucher and Lee Powers. Atlanta, Ga., Oct. 5–8, 1963.

"Report of the Second Administrative Institute: Medical School-Teaching Hospital Relations." Report of the Twelfth AAMC Institute of the Association of American Medical Colleges. ed. George A. Wolf, Jr., Ray E. Brown, and Robert M. Bucher. Miami Beach, Fla., Dec. 6–9, 1964.

"Medical Ventures and the University: New Values and New Validities." Report of the Thirteenth AAMC Institute, Third Institute on Administration. ed. Douglas M. Knight and E. Shepley Nourse. Bal Harbour, Fla., Dec. 12–15, 1965.

23. Kendall, P. "Relationship Between Medical Educators and Medical Practitioners: Sources of Strain and Occasions for Cooperation in Educators and Practitioners as Factors in Medical and Health Care," *Medical Education and Medical Care: Interactions and Prospects.* Evanston, Ill.: AAMC, 1961.

24. Somers, A. "Conflict, Accommodation, and Progress: Some Socioeconomic Observations on Medical Education and the Prac-

ticing Profession," in *Medical Education and Medical Care: Interactions and Prospects*. Evanston, Ill.: AAMC, 1961.

25. *Bulletin of the Association of American Medical Colleges 1:2* (Nov. 14, 1966).

26. Ebert, R. "The Role of the Medical School in Planning the Health Care System." *J. Med. Educ. 42:*481 (June 1967).

27. Somers, A. R., and H. M. Somers. "Grantsmanship and Stewardship: A Public View." *Public Health Reports 80:*660 (August 1965).

28. Harris, R. *A Sacred Trust*. New York: New American Library, 1966.

29. Carter, R. *The Doctor Business*. Garden City, N. Y.: Doubleday, 1958.

30. *Medical Economics 42:*103–107 (Dec. 13, 1965).

31. "A Study of the Quality of Hospital Care Secured by a Sample of Teamster Family Members in New York City." A Joint Project of Teamsters Joint Council No. 16 and Management Hospitalization Trust Fund, Montefiore Hospital and Columbia University School of Public Health and Administrative Medicine, 1964.

32. Baehr, G. "Medical Care: Old Goals and New Horizons." The 1965 Michael M. Davis Lecture, Center for Health Administration Studies, Graduate School of Business, University of Chicago, 1965.

33. Morison, R. "Some Illnesses of Mental Health (The Alan Gregg Lecture, 1964)." *J. Med. Educ. 39:*985 (1964).

34. Collen, M. F. "Periodic Health Examinations Using an Automated Multitest Laboratory." *JAMA 195:*142 (1962).

35. "Professional Standards for Medical Groups and Standards for Medical Group Centers." Health Insurance Plan for Greater New York. October 1964.

36. "The Graduate Education of Physicians." The Report of the Citizens' Commission on Graduate Medical Education. Chicago: AMA, August 1966.

37. Sodeman, W. A. "Responsibilities of Medicine to the Basic Sciences," *JAMA 193:*122–124 (Aug. 16, 1965).

Chapter 3. The Consumer Revolution:
Translating Knowledge into Programs
(1960–1968)

1. *Medical Care Studies and Family Income*. National Center for Health Statistics, Chronic Illness and Disability. Department of Health, Education and Welfare. Washington, D. C., 1964.

2. Seifert, V. D. and J. S. Johnstone. "Meeting the Emergency Department Crisis." *Hospitals, JAHA 40*:55 (Nov. 1, 1966).

3. Lashof, J. C. and M. H. Lepper. "Health and Medical Care in Poverty Areas of Chicago." *Presbyterian—St. Luke's Hospital Med. Bull. 5*:188 (October 1966).

4. Somers, H. M. "Financing of Medical Care." *New Eng. J. Med. 275*:702 (Sept. 29, 1966).

5. "Building America's Health: Condensation of the Report of the President's Commission on the Health Needs of the Nation." Raleigh, N. C.: Health Publications Institute, Inc., 1953.

6. Mayo, L. W. *A Report of the President's Panel on a Proposed Program for National Action to Combat Mental Retardation.* Washington, D. C.: U.S. Government Printing Office, 1963.

7. Kennedy, J. F. *Message from the President of the United States Relative to a Health Program.* Feb. 27, 1962. 87th Congress, 2nd Session, House of Representatives, Document No. 347.

8. Russell, J. M. "New Federal Regional Medical Programs." *New Eng. J. of Med. 275*:309 (1966).

9. A National Program to Conquer Heart Disease, Cancer and Stroke. Washington, D. C.: U.S. Government Printing Office, vol. 1, December, 1964; vol. 2, February 1965.

10. Miller, G. E. "Medical Care: Its Social and Organizational Aspects: The Continuing Education of Physicians." *New Eng. J. Med. 269*:295–299 (1963).

11. May, C. "Selling Drugs by 'Educating' Physicians." *J. Med. Educ. 36*:1–23 (1961).

12. Dunlop, J. T. "The Capacity of the United States to Provide and Finance Expanding Health Services." *Bull. N. Y. Acad. Med. 41*: 1325 (December 1965).

13. James, G. Address to Conference of Community Leaders on New Health Programs, Albany, N. Y., December 8, 1966. Duplicated.

14. Hearings before the Special Subcommittee on Investigation of Dept. of Health, Education and Welfare of the Committee on Interstate and Foreign Commerce, House of Representatives, 89th Congress, 2nd Session. Ser. No. 89–42. Washington, D. C.: U.S. Government Printing Office, 1966, p. 1, 2.

15. Report of the Special Subcommittee on Investigation of the Dept. of Health, Education, and Welfare of the Committee on Interstate and Foreign Commerce, House of Representatives, 89th Congress, 2nd Session, U.S. Government Printing Office, Washington, Oct. 13, 1966, p. 28.

16. Comprehensive Neighborhood Health Services Programs, Office of Economic Opportunity, Washington, D. C., February 1967.

17. Bamberger, L. "Health Care and Poverty: What Are the Dimensions of the Problem from the Community's Point of View?" *Bull. N. Y. Acad. Med. 42*:1140–49 (December 1966).

18. Yerby, A. "The Disadvantaged and Health Care (Presentation at White House Conference on Health, Nov. 1965)." *Am. J. Public Health 56*:5 (January 1966).

19. *Consumer Issues '66: A Report to the President from the Consumer Advisory Council.* Washington, D. C., June 12, 1966.

Chapter 4. Some Conceptual and Programmatic Issues Facing Medicine

1. Menninger, K. *The Vital Balance: The Life Process in Mental Health and Illness.* New York: Viking Press, 1963.

2. Stone, A., and Gloria Onque. *Longitudinal Studies of Child Personality: Abstracts with Index.* Cambridge, Mass.: Harvard University Press, 1959.

3. Miller, S. M. "Solving the Urban Dilemma in Health Care: More Poverty, Greater Demand for Public Services, Reduced Financial Resources, and Fragmentation of Services," *Bull. N. Y. Acad. Med. 42*:1150–56 (December 1966).

4. Roemer, M. I., and M. Shain. *Hospital Utilization under Insurance.* Chicago: American Hospital Association, 1959.

5. London, M., and R. M. Sigmond. "Are We Building Too Many Hospital Beds?" *The Modern Hosp. 96*:59 (January 1961).

6. "Improving the Opportunities and Achievements of Children of the Poor." Report of Planning Committee, Project Head Start, Office of Economic Opportunity, February 1965.

7. Richmond, J. B. "How Long, Oh Lord, How Long?" *Am. J. of Orthopsychiat. 37*:4 (1957).

8. Cope, O., and J. Zacharias. *Medical Education Reconsidered.* Philadelphia & Montreal: Lippincott, 1966.

9. Cope, O. "The Future of Medical Education." *Harper's Magazine 235*:98 (October 1967).

10. Fein, R. *The Doctor Shortage: An Economic Diagnosis.* Washington, D. C.: The Brookings Institution, May 1967.

11. Darley, W., and A. R. Somers. "Medicine, Money and Manpower: The Challenge to Professional Education." "I. The Affluent New Health-Care Economy," *New Eng. J. Med. 276*:1234–38 (June 1, 1967). "II. Opportunity for New Excellence," *New Eng. J. Med. 276*:1291–96 (June 8, 1967). "III. Increasing Personnel," *New Eng. J.*

Med. 276:1414–23 (June 22, 1967). "IV. New Training for New Needs," *New Eng. J. Med. 276*:1471–78 (June 29, 1967).

12. Nelson, B. "Unplugging the Muted Trumpet: Senate Says —NIH, Blow Your Horn." *Science 154*:491 (Oct. 28, 1966).

13. "The Advancement of Knowledge for the Nation's Health." A Report to the President on the Research Programs of the National Institutes of Health, Department of Health, Education and Welfare, July, 1967.

14. Handler, P. "Academic Science and the Federal Government." *Science 157*:1140–46 (Sept. 8, 1967).

15. White, K. L. "Primary Medical Care for Families: Organization and Evaluation." *New Eng. J. Med. 277*:847 (Oct. 19, 1967).

16. Borgatta, E. F. "Research Problems in Evaluation of Health Service Demonstrations." *Milbank Mem. Fund Quarterly 44*:182 (October 1966).

17. Gould, S. "The Modern University: Concerns for the Future." *Science 155*:1511 (Mar. 24, 1967).

Chapter 5. Approaches to Complexity

1. "Report of the First Institute on Clinical Teaching." Report of the Sixth Teaching Institute of the Association of American Medical Colleges. ed. Helen H. Gee and J. B. Richmond. Swampscott, Mass., Oct. 7–11, 1958.

2. Binger, C. *The Doctor's Job.* New York: Norton, 1945.

3. Gregg, A. *Multiple Causation and Organismic and Integrative Approaches to Medical Education.* Washington, D. C.: Conference on Psychiatric Education, American Psychiatric Association, 1951.

4. Richmond, J. B., and S. L. Lustman. "Total Health: A Conceptual Visual Aid," *J. Med. Educ. 29*:23 (1954).

5. Coggeshall, L. T. "New Directions in Medical Education." Address presented at Brown University, Nov. 3, 1966.

6. Sanazaro, P. J. "Emerging Patterns in Medical Education." *Mayo Clinic Proc. 42*:777 (December 1967).

7. Oppenheimer, R. "Tree of Knowledge." *Harper's Mag.* (October 1958), p. 55.

8. Ebert, R. "The Role of the Medical School in Planning the Health Care System." *J. Med. Educ. 42*:481 (June 1967).

9. Fein, R. *The Doctor Shortage: An Economic Diagnosis.* Washington, D. C.: The Brookings Institution, May 1967.

10. *Report of the National Advisory Commission on Health*

Manpower. Vol. I, Washington, D. C.: U.S. Government Printing Office, November 1967.

11. Langer, E. "Who Makes our Health Policy?" *Physicians' Forum* (June 1967), p. 5.

Index

American Academy of General Practice, 61

American Cancer Society, 71

American Foundation Studies in Government: *American Medicine: Expert Testimony Out of Court* (1937), 16, 19

American Heart Association, 71

American Hospital Association, 71

American Medical Association (AMA): Council on Medical Education, 2, 4–5, 6, 10, 20; report of Committee on Social Insurance (1917), 8; Board of Trustees, 8, 11, 22, 51, 52, 59, 87; on public health service programs, 8–9, 15–16, 29, 50–54, 59–60, 76–77; Freymann on, 9; political structure of, 9, 15; policy struggle in, 9–10; organizational structure of, 10–11, 23; political lobbying of, 11, 50, 71, 81; House of Delegates, 11, 86; opposes report of "Committee of 430," 18–20; speciality section of, 21; individual practitioners' feelings about, 23; its attitude toward NIH, 29; *vs.* Medicare, 44, 53, 68, 79–80; public relations staff of, 50–52; opposes Wagner-Murray-Dingle Bill, 50; *vs.* vendor payment enactments, 50, 53, 54, 56, 78; supports Kerr-Mills Bill, 53, 80; opinion by Supreme Court, 57–58; opposes report of Commission on Heart Disease, Cancer, and Stroke, 71; Reference Committee on Insurance and Medical Service *B* (Report AA), 87; report of Ad Hoc Committee on Education for Family Practice, 88–90, 98

American Public Health Association, 23, 56

Appalachian Regional Council, 82

Association of American Medical Colleges (AAMC): standard curriculum of, 4, 6; collaborates with AMA on accreditation, 10; supports institutionalized medicine, 23; membership of, 39, 40, 41; Russell on, 39–40; lack of leadership in, 39–41, 44–47; reorganization study committee of, 40–41; its reaction to Coggeshall Report, 41–44; work of Darley in, 44–45; changes headquarters, 45; work of Berry in, 45; Executive Council, 81

Associations of Medical School Departmental Chairmen, 47

Bellaire (Ohio) Medical Group: court cases of, 58

Berry, George P., 45

Berson, Robert C., 40

Blue Cross, 54

Blue Shield, 54

Boston: practitioners in poverty areas, 64

Bureau of the Budget: cost-sharing

Gregg, Alan: on disease causations, 114–115

Group Health Association of America, 23, 57

Group practice, *see* Institutionalized medicine

Harris, Richard, 50

Harvard Medical School: Flexner on, 3–4; *The New England Journal of Medicine* on, 7

Health, Education and Welfare Department (HEW): Children's Bureau of, 15, 75, 86, 94; growth of, 29; medical school administrators' appeal to, 34

Health Insurance Plan of Greater New York, 58

Health Professions Assistance Act (1963), 81

Health service programs: AMA's stand on health insurance, 7–8, 15–16, 18–20, 29, 50–53; recommended by Committee on the Costs of Medical Care, 11–14; history of, 14, 57; in USPHS, 14, 15; in Children's Bureau and Welfare Administration, 15; report of "Committee of 430" on, 16–18; effect of research programs on, 53, 108–109; hospitalization plans of, 54; preventive care programs, 55–57; protected by courts, 57–58; in Kaiser Industries, 58; Health Insurance Plan of Greater New York, 58; of United Mine Workers, 58–59; mental health and retardation programs of, 69–70; Commission on Heart Disease, Cancer, and Stroke, 70–73 *passim;* possible future developments of, 95–96; community health centers *vs.* hospitals, 97–98; society's responsibility in, 104–107; importance of preprofessional education in, 107–108; need for national strategy in, 109–110; future

financing of, 109; evaluation difficulties in, 113–116. *See also* Congress, health legislation in; Medicare, Social Security Act; Vendor payments

Hill-Burton Bill, 67–68, 97

Hospitals, public: deterioration of, 63–64; increasing use of emergency rooms in, 64, 67; Hill-Burton Bill for construction of, 67–68, 97; their role in institutionalized medicine and research programs, 96–97; Comprehensive Health Planning Act (1965), 97; *vs.* community health centers, 97–98; financial crisis of, 99–100; utilization of, 99–101; management problems of, 101–103

House Committee on Interstate and Foreign Commerce: promotes study of health, education, and welfare (1965), 82

Hubbard, William N., 40

Hudson, Charles L.: on inadequacy of health services for the poor, 86

Illinois: internship requirements for licensure in, 20

Institutionalized medicine (group practice): effects of World War II on, 23; growth of, 46; report of Citizens' Commission on Graduate Medical Education, 59–60; family care plan (1965), 83–85; Yerby on clinics, 85–86; new emphasis on generalist-specialists, 88–90; related to community health programs, 94–98; role of hospital in, 96–97; related to research, 119

Internship: early statutory specifications of, 20; accrediting process of, 20–21

Jefferson, Thomas, 119

Jencks, C.: on higher education, 36

Osteopathy, schools of: present status of, 5

Pennsylvania: Flexner on medical school, 3–4; internship requirements for licensure in, 20

Perera, George A., 40

Presidential Panel on Mental Retardation, 51–52

President's Commission on the Health Needs of the Nation (1951), 67

President's Consumer Advisory Council: report on health services (1966), 87, 90

Project Head Start (Office of Economic Opportunity): purpose of, 75; public response to, 75–76; report of Planning Committee of, 105–106

Public Health Service, 29, 68

Regional Medical Programs for Heart Disease, Cancer, Stroke, and Related Diseases, 82, 98, 105

Research: growth of, 10; federal funding program in, 28–33 passim; problems related to grants in, 31–38 passim; effect of grants on outpatient care and public health services, 47–49, 53, 108–109; role of hospital in, 96–97; related to institutionalized medicine, 119

"Research in the Service of Man" conference, 27

Residency: for specialized training, 21; effect of depression on, 21–22

Rockefeller Foundation: General Education Board's medical grants (1910–1928), 3

Rogers, Paul G.: on national health problems, 82

Russell, John: on AAMC, 39–40, 45

Sanazaro, Paul: on possible future medical education, 117

Shadid, Michael, 57

Shannon, James, 38

Sigerist, Henry, 21

Social Security Act (1936): recognition of health service needs, 15; maternal and child health services, 15, 75; early medical reaction to, 24. See also Medicare; Vendor payments

Society of Internal Medicine, 55

Sodeman, William, 61

Somers, Anne, 23; "Conflict, Accommodation, and Progress: Some Socioeconomic Observations on Medical Education and the Practicing Profession," 46–47

Somers, Herman: on objectives of health insurance programs, 64–65, 66

Special Subcommittee on HEW Investigation (1965), 82

Specialization: growth of, 9–10, 20–21; Advisory Board on, 21–22; hospital training in, 21; influence of World War II on, 22–24; effect on comprehensive medical care, 83

Sputnik I: effect of on educational achievements, 116

Stevenson, Adlai, 50

Supreme Court: AMA vs. U.S., 57–58

Truman, Harry S.: interested in medical care programs, 29, 50, 67

Turner, Thomas B.: on AAMC and Coggeshall Report, 43–44

United Auto Workers, 59

United Mine Workers: Health and Welfare Fund of, 58–59

United States Public Health Service (USPHS): growth of, 14; National Health Survey of, 8, 14, 101